EASY EXERCISES

— *for* —

PREGNANCY

Janet Balaskas

Photographs by Anthea Sieveking

FRANCES LINCOLN

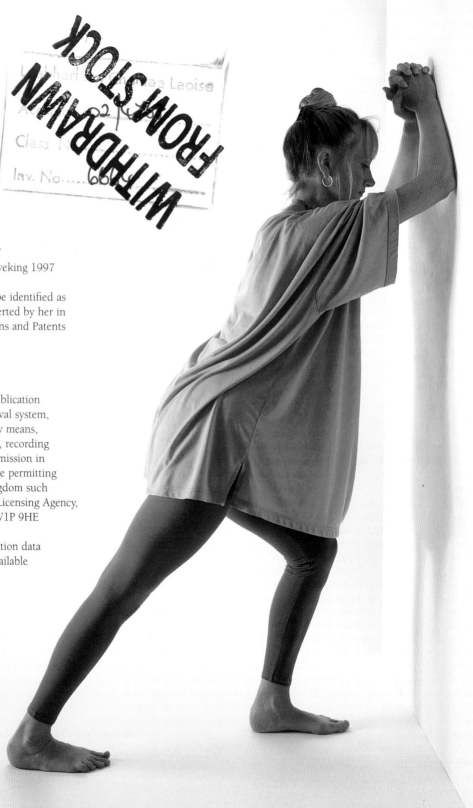

Frances Lincoln Limited
4 Torriano Mews
Torriano Avenue
London NW5 2RZ

Easy Exercises for Pregnancy
Copyright © Frances Lincoln 1997
Text copyright © Janet Balaskas 1997
Photographs copyright © Anthea Sieveking 1997

First Frances Lincoln edition: 1997

British Library Cataloguing in Publication data
A catalogue record for this book is available
from the British Library.

ISBN 0 7112 1048 9

Set in Berkeley Old Style
Printed in Hong Kong by
Kwong Fat Offset Printing Co. Ltd

9 8 7 6 5 4 3 2

CONTENTS

THE BENEFITS OF EXERCISE

Choosing to introduce a programme of easy exercises into your daily life is a very positive decision. This is particularly so while you are pregnant and have the challenges of carrying your growing baby, giving birth and the postnatal months ahead of you.

This book teaches you how to use your body positively. This will make a tremendous difference to your health and the way you feel while you are pregnant. It can also empower you to cope well with your labour and birth, to recover quickly afterwards and to enjoy good health and energy when caring for your baby.

You can use this exercise programme whether this is your first, second or subsequent baby, or if you are carrying twins. Generally, the movements and positions they involve are helpful for women who have back pain, sciatica and most of the common problems that can occur in pregnancy, although it is always wise to check with your midwife or doctor and show them this book before you start. It is a good idea to go for a gentle walk or swim two or three times a week in addition to doing some of these exercises

on a daily basis. This should be all you need to be fit and healthy throughout your pregnancy.

The exercises are especially designed for pregnancy and are based on more than 15 years' experience of teaching pregnant women. It is very important that exercise is not strenuous. This is because your heart and lungs are already working at increased levels in pregnancy, which is itself a natural kind of aerobic exercise. The last thing you need is an aerobic 'workout' on top of that. And yet you do need to exercise your body sensibly and to keep fit.

If you follow the instructions carefully you will find that the exercises in this book are easy to do, as well as safe for you and your baby. They are effective and relaxing and yet not strenuous in any way.

Many of the exercises can fit in with your daily routine. For example, you can sit in the tailor position (page 26) for a few minutes while watching television, or do a forward bend (page 41) while waiting for the kettle to boil. However, if you can make the time, it is beneficial to set aside 30–60 minutes a day especially for practising the exercises. This will give you an opportunity to unwind and relax each day and to pay attention to yourself and the vital work you are doing in nourishing your baby. This is particularly helpful if you are working in pregnancy. It will help you to cope better with even the busiest lifestyle. If this is your second or a subsequent baby, this may be the only time you really have for yourself to devote to recharging your energy and focusing on the new baby.

Increasing energy

Many women complain about tiredness and exhaustion in pregnancy. This is not surprising as your body is working harder than usual to protect and nourish your baby. However, feeling tired is also caused by stagnant or blocked energy due to a lack of suitable exercise or poor posture. Your energy level can improve dramatically when you start to practise a few simple exercises on a regular basis. You may also find that you are sleeping better at night!

I always notice, after an exercise class, that mothers who arrived feeling exhausted are more energized and refreshed by the time they leave. The effect is cumulative too, so that exercising regularly, in the right way, can transform the months ahead from a time of discomfort and indisposition to one in which you feel healthy, strong and energetic.

Improving posture

Now that you are carrying a baby your posture is more important than ever. Our modern lifestyle often results in poor postural habits which can affect us in pregnancy. For example, watching television lying back on the sofa with your feet up on the coffee table may seem relaxing but it slows down the circulation of blood to the placenta and could be encouraging your baby into a less advantageous position for the birth, especially in late pregnancy. In fact it is much better to sit up straight with your back well supported, or else to lie on your side or to relax leaning forwards over a beanbag.

As you practise the exercises in this book you will also be learning how to position and use your body positively when going about your daily life. This includes when you are standing, walking, sitting, working at a desk, resting and relaxing, watching television or sleeping. Not only will you feel much better, but your baby will benefit from a better supply of nutrients and oxygen and you will be doing your best to help your baby move into a good position for labour and birth.

Encouraging flexibility and suppleness

The exercises in this book are all natural movements our bodies are designed to make with ease. However, because of the way we live, there are certain movements we do not make very often and they can become difficult to do. Squatting or kneeling are good examples of this. Young children use these positions with ease all the time but, as adults, we rarely make such movements. As a result our joints stiffen and muscles shorten so that, when we try to squat or kneel, we may encounter resistance and pain. However, flexibility and muscle tone can be improved and even restored by safe and sensible exercise.

During pregnancy your body becomes softer and more pliable than usual; this softening is caused by changes in your hormones, and because of this you can improve your flexibility much more easily. In this book you are guided to do this in an easy, gentle way, using the support of cushions, a wall, a beanbag, a chair or a stool, to allow for gradual release of tension, helped along by your breathing. This is enjoyable and painless and means that you can make the most of the changes of pregnancy to improve your general physical condition. These benefits will last if you keep on exercising postnatally.

Improving the flexibility of your pelvic joints, hips, knees and ankles will make it possible for you to feel more comfortable while using supported upright positions during labour and when you give birth.

Good breathing

The breathing exercise on page 12 teaches you to be aware of your natural breathing rhythm. Then the instructions for each exercise always include this awareness, so that you learn to focus on the wave-like rise and fall of the breath to help you relax and release tension in each position. Once you get used to doing this, you will find that your breathing flows effortlessly and your overall lung capacity improves. Your body will respond by becoming looser and more flexible, and this, combined with good posture, means better circulation both for yourself and also for your baby. So you will be helping your baby to breathe better too, as well as to get more vital nutrients needed for healthy growth and development, while enhancing your own vitality and health.

In labour, being able to focus on the natural rhythm of your breathing will give you a powerful tool for managing the pain during contractions. This will enable you to relax and surrender to the work your uterus is doing: opening and bringing your baby to birth. If you choose to go through labour without pain-killers this is invaluable. It may also be helpful if you do opt for some intervention. Even if you have a caesarean section, knowing how to concentrate on your breathing and relax can make a big difference. Being able to focus on your spontaneous breathing rhythm during contractions in labour is more effective than learning breathing techniques, especially when you are free to move and choose the most comfortable position at the same time.

Becoming 'grounded'

You will notice that I often use the word 'grounded' in this book. This is because the sort of exercise I recommend makes you aware of the power of the earth underneath you and how the force of gravity influences your posture at all times. As you get the feel of this you will feel more 'grounded' or more in touch with the earth. This gives you a feeling of physical support and balance and, at the same time, a sense of emotional calm and equilibrium. You will find that 'being grounded' in the lower part of your body enables you to relax and release tension in your spine, neck and shoulders, to avoid headaches and to cope much better with stress.

This is also going to be very useful in labour when you will find that you can release the pain by breathing into the ground. There is a constant exchange during contractions in which the earth seems to absorb pain and give back fresh energy. Being 'grounded' helps you to stay calm and relaxed as well as nourished by this help from the earth, leaving your upper body free to relax and expand into the space around you.

A positive pregnancy

I believe that it is essential to do something in pregnancy which reminds you every day that there is a miracle taking place in your body. These exercises make you feel great. They let you know that everything is going well. They help you to have confidence in your body and to approach labour optimistically and without fear. You also have the satisfaction of knowing that you are doing your best for yourself and your baby, and making the most of this wonderful time in your life.

EXERCISING ON YOUR OWN

Exercising on your own is a health-giving habit to develop that brings many benefits into your life. The most valuable exercise time is when you are alone and can concentrate on what you are doing undisturbed for 30–60 minutes. So the first thing that you need to do is to create the time.

Space and equipment

You will need a warm, uncluttered space with a free wall and some basic equipment. This includes a simple, straight-backed chair and a low stool (about 25cm/10in high). If you can manage to invest in a beanbag you will find it invaluable. Otherwise three or four very large cushions will do. You will need a few small cushions or pillows as well. Some of the exercises suggest using a firm bolster and these can be obtained from a futon shop. However, a rolled-up sleeping bag or two blankets rolled up into a sausage shape make good substitutes. You will need to work on a soft surface such as a carpet or rug or to place a folded blanket underneath you.

If you sit for long periods at work then use an adjustable kneeling stool such as the one on page 30 or a chair with good back support and a seat that slopes downwards, or put two cushions on the seat so that your pelvis is slightly higher than your knees (page 31).

Clothing

It is important to be comfortable while you exercise so wear a big loose T-shirt and some comfortable leggings, loose trousers or shorts. It is best to have bare feet when you do these exercises.

To begin with

When you start, read through all the instructions first, including the boxed sections headed REMEMBER. If the exercise recommends closing your eyes, then read the text again before you try. Do not worry if you cannot remember all the suggestions at first. You will, with practice, and eventually all you will need to remember what to do is to glance at the picture. Work through each section gradually, doing as little or as much as you want to at a time. Always begin the

BREATHING and BABY AWARENESS (see pages 12–13) and end with a relaxation exercise (see pages 54–57).

You can do all of the exercises, or just some of them, varying your choice through the week. In addition to following this programme of exercises at home on your own, you will benefit by going for a walk in the open air two or three times a week, or doing some gentle swimming .

Aches and pains

Minor aches and pains may very well improve once you begin to practise these exercises regularly. However, if you have back pain or sciatica, or any other more serious problems, consulting an osteopath who specializes in treating pregnant women is a good idea (see USEFUL ADDRESSES on page 192). Show your practitioner this book before you start this programme so that he or she can suggest which exercises if any might be especially beneficial or should be avoided.

Always avoid or modify any exercise which causes you pain or discomfort beyond 'beginners stiffness'. After a week or two the exercises should be easy to do and completely comfortable.

Many women feel wonderful in pregnancy, but some do not and feel sick or exhausted, especially in the early months. If you are suffering like this, start the exercises very slowly, without doing too much at first, and stop if you are uneasy or any particular exercise does not feel comfortable. In time exercising should help you to feel much better, but begin gradually, always respecting what your body is telling you. Remember this is not a 'workout'.

Listen to your body

Learning from a teacher or a book can work very well but, ultimately, your own body is your best guide to sensible exercise. Listen to what your body tells you at all times – stop if you have had enough, leave out an exercise if you do not feel comfortable with it, or stay in it for longer than suggested if you want to. Always be kind and gentle to your body and avoid using force or pushing yourself beyond your limits. You want to end up feeling relaxed and energized, and above all to enjoy yourself while doing these exercises.

BREATHING

This exercise helps you focus awareness on your natural breathing rhythm. You can use this awareness while doing all the exercises in this book, and also during labour or when breastfeeding your baby.

1 Sit on the floor on the edge of a small cushion. Cross your legs comfortably and tuck one or two cushions under each knee so that your legs feel well supported.

2 Release your lower back downwards so that your weight settles into your pelvis. Then gently lengthen your spine from the waistline up towards the top of your head, without arching your lower back.

3 Lengthen the back of your neck by lowering your chin slightly towards your chest. Relax your shoulders and let your arms hang loosely by your sides with your hands resting softly on your knees.

4 Close your eyes and allow your eyelids and the muscles of your face to become soft and relaxed. Loosen your jaw. Let your awareness go to your breathing.

5 Breathe evenly in your natural rhythm, simply noticing each time you breathe out and breathe in.

6 Continue observing your breathing, noticing a little pause at the end of each out breath, before the next breath comes in. Relax, take your time and continue like this for up to three minutes, then slowly open your eyes and relax.

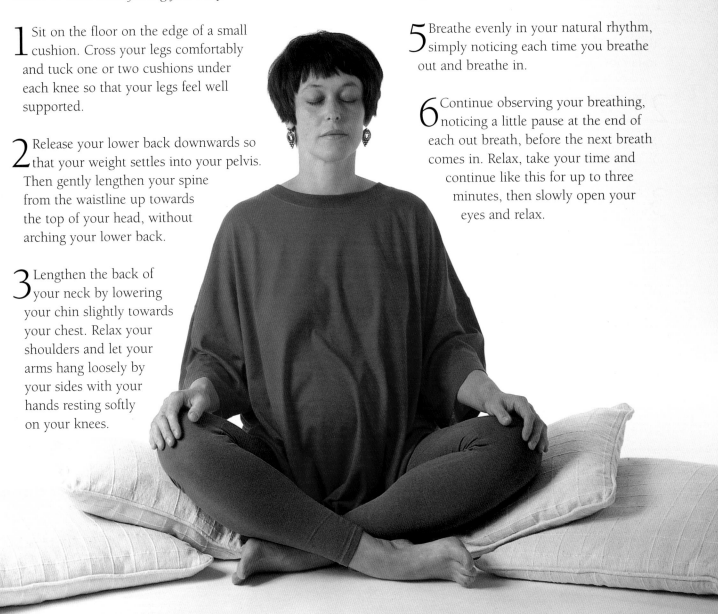

BABY AWARENESS

Sitting quietly and focusing on the rhythm of your breathing helps you to be more aware of the presence of your baby. These 'special times' you share together are precious moments in your pregnancy.

1 Seated comfortably upright with legs crossed, place your hands softly on your lower belly to cradle your baby. Close your eyes and relax the back of your neck, allowing your head to fall forward comfortably.

2 Bring your awareness to your breathing rhythm and then to the presence of your baby inside. Notice whether your baby is moving or lying still.

3 Now imagine what your baby is feeling and hearing; the soft sensations of warm fluid caressing the skin and the reassuring rhythm of your heart beating. Be aware of the deep connection between you and your baby and, if you like, talk to your baby inwardly.

4 Spend the next few minutes breathing comfortably and simply relaxing with your baby. When you are ready, slowly bring your awareness back to your breathing, your body and the room around you, and then open your eyes.

Remember
Above all, do not try! Allow the breath to flow, inhaling and exhaling through your nose as usual, without trying to breathe in any special way. (If your nose is blocked, breathe through your mouth.)

TOES AND HEELS

The easy movements here and in CIRCLING FEET *opposite improve the circulation to and from your legs, so try to do them every day.*

1 Sit on the floor with your lower back supported by a wall, or sit on the edge of a small cushion and relax your lower back downwards, then lengthen your spine. Stretch your legs out in front of you with your heels about 30cm/12in apart.

2 Relax your arms and shoulders and rest your hands on your thighs. Close your eyes for a moment before you start and feel the way the backs of your legs contact the floor. Breathe evenly in your normal rhythm.

3 Open your eyes and look at your feet. Separate and wiggle your toes and relax them.

4 First point your toes away from you and then, as shown, extend your heels, stretching them away from you as you flex your toes towards you.

5 Alternating these two movements, first toes and then heels, repeat ten times.

CIRCLING FEET

1 Sit against a wall or on the edge of a cushion as for the TOES AND HEELS exercise opposite.

2 Spread your legs a little wider so that your heels are about 60–90cm/2–3ft apart. Make big, wide circles with your feet, rolling them inwards towards the centre from the ankles, and repeat 10 times.

3 Now reverse the movement, rolling the feet outwards away from the centre.

4 Repeat the inward and outward circles ten times and then relax your feet.

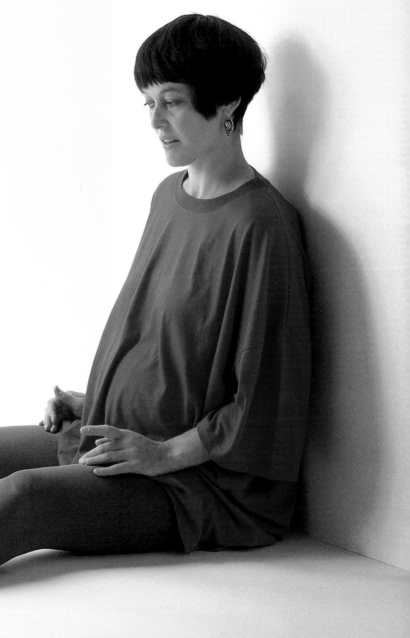

NECK ROLL

Slow rolling movements combined with easy breathing gently release tension in the neck, jaw and head.

1 Sit on the floor on the edge of a small cushion. Cross your legs comfortably and place a cushion or two under each knee so that your legs feel well supported.

2 Release your lower back towards the ground, so that your weight settles into your pelvis. Gently lengthen your spine so that you grow tall from the waist up towards your head without arching your lower back.

3 Relax your shoulders, let your arms fall softly by your sides, and place your hands on your knees. Loosen your jaw and breathe evenly in your normal rhythm.

4 Keeping your back upright, slowly release your head forwards to relax the muscles at the back of your neck.

5 Breathe evenly and begin to roll your head very slowly around in big soft circles, releasing any tension in your neck. Continue the movement until you have completed three circles and come back to the centre.

6 Pause for a second or two, be aware of your breathing, and repeat in the opposite direction.

7 Slowly raise your head and return to the starting position.

SHOULDER RELEASE

This is an exercise to loosen and relax your shoulders, and calm and 'centre' you as you end with the prayer position.

1 Sit relaxed and do steps 1–3 of the NECK ROLL exercise opposite.

2 Roll your shoulders backwards, making easy circular movements. Repeat this slowly up to ten times.

3 When your shoulders feel nice and loose, end by dropping them back and down, creating a lovely open feeling across the front of the chest.

4 Place the palms of your hands together softly and close your eyes. Focus on your breathing and enjoy a few minutes of inner calm. Feel how this movement brings your awareness within to your inner centre.

5 Release your hands and open your eyes.

Remember

The movements for NECK ROLL and SHOULDER RELEASE should be made slowly and softly. When you sit upright, always release your lower back downwards first and then gently feel your spine lengthen from the ground up towards the sky. There should be no arching or feeling of pulling up at the back of the waist.

PALM STRETCH

This is a way to release tension in the fingers, hands and wrists, and improve circulation to and from the hands. Repeat it three or four times.

1 Kneel on the floor on a soft surface with a long cushion or bolster between your knees. Release the base of your spine downwards. Relax your shoulders and arms and link your fingers.

2 Bend your elbows and turn your hands so that your palms are facing outwards. Extend your arms and stretch your fingers gently.

3 Breathe evenly, keeping your shoulders relaxed, and hold for about three cycles of your breathing rhythm.

4 Bend your elbows and turn your palms to face inwards. Then unclasp your hands and shake them loosely from the wrists to relax them.

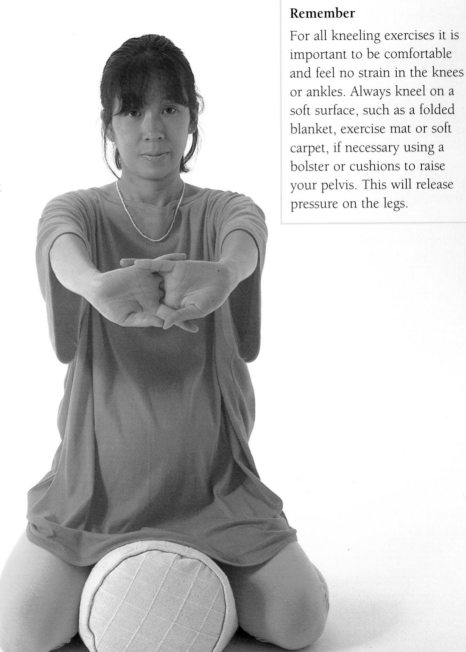

Remember
For all kneeling exercises it is important to be comfortable and feel no strain in the knees or ankles. Always kneel on a soft surface, such as a folded blanket, exercise mat or soft carpet, if necessary using a bolster or cushions to raise your pelvis. This will release pressure on the legs.

ARMS RAISED

This exercise releases tension in your shoulders with a sense of gentle lengthening upwards from a stable base in the pelvis. In late pregnancy it can help to make more space for the baby, and relieve pressure under the ribs.

Remember

If your fingers or wrists are swollen and hurt when you turn the palms out, try easier versions of both this and the previous exercise keeping your elbows slightly bent. It is also important to keep your weight centred in your pelvis when you make these movements, and to avoid any arching or pulling up in the back of your waist.

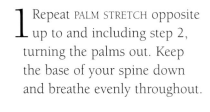

1 Repeat PALM STRETCH opposite up to and including step 2, turning the palms out. Keep the base of your spine down and breathe evenly throughout.

2 On an exhalation, slowly bring your arms up over your head with your elbows slightly bent, and keep releasing the base of your spine gently downwards as your arms come up.

3 Very gently, and without arching your lower back, straighten your elbows, opening your palms towards the sky.

4 Hold for just a few seconds, and then, on an exhalation, slowly lower your arms and unclasp your hands.

5 Shake your hands softly from the wrists and then relax.

SHOULDER RELEASE

This movement improves the flexibility of the shoulders, relieves pressure under the ribs and improves breathing.

1 Kneel on the floor on a soft surface with a long cushion or bolster between your legs. Sit back on your heels and relax with your feet turning inwards. Release your lower back downwards and settle into your pelvis.

2 Slowly raise one arm up over your head. Bend your elbow and reach down your spine with your fingers without straining.

3 Now raise the other arm and catch hold of your elbow, easing it gently towards the ceiling without pulling. Breathe evenly and hold the position for about three cycles of the breath.

4 Release both arms, rest and repeat on the other side.

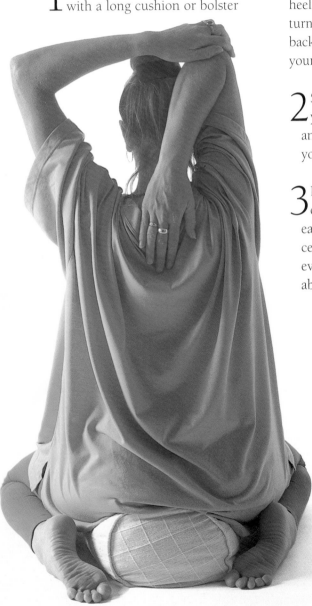

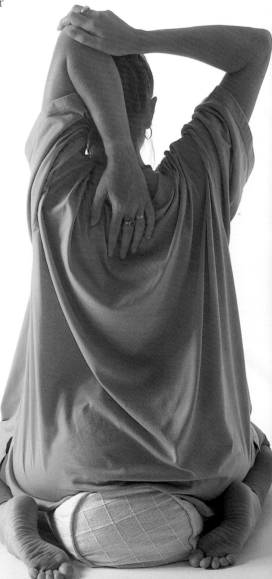

Remember
Allow the release to take place slowly as you breathe. Keep your lower back down and your neck relaxed.

SHOULDER STRETCH

This movement is lovely to practise in pregnancy, and is also helpful postnatally to release tension in the shoulders after carrying or feeding your baby.

1 Kneel on the floor on a soft surface with your knees about 30cm/12in away from a wall. Place a long cushion between your legs if you like.

2 Spread your knees apart and turn your feet in towards the centre. Sit back on your heels, drop your lower back and settle into your pelvis.

3 Raise both arms gently above your head, keeping the base of your spine down. Lean forwards slowly from your hips and reach up the wall, placing your palms about 30cm/12in apart.

4 With your arms straight, drop your weight down into your hips, curling your lower back round softly towards your heels.

5 Now relax between your shoulders until you feel a gentle stretch in your shoulders and upper arms. Breathe evenly and hold the position for about three cycles of the breathing rhythm.

6 Release your arms and curl up slowly, first dropping your lower back down towards your feet. Roll your shoulders gently backwards a few times and then repeat one more time.

Remember
Keep your lower back and pelvis down. Release your tailbone towards your feet throughout to avoid arching your back. Breathe comfortably in your normal rhythm.

SPREADING OUT

This movement gives you a feeling of being wide as well as long in your upper body, so it makes plenty of space for your baby. You can practise it like this, sitting on the floor, or when you are seated upright on a chair, perhaps at the table or your desk, to increase your awareness of your posture throughout the day.

1 Sit in the starting position given on page 16. You might like to refold your legs with the other one in front. Release your lower back downwards and then lengthen your spine gently from the back of the waist up to the top of your head.

2 Extend your arms sideways and touch the ground very lightly with your fingertips. Breathe evenly and, making tiny 'flying' movements in slow motion, allow your hands to lift slowly off the ground.

3 Open your arms softly outwards on either side of your body, like a pair of beautiful wings unfolding. Slowly continue lifting your arms until they reach the height of your shoulders.

4 Keep your shoulders and wrists relaxed. Hold for a few seconds and breathe evenly in your normal rhythm.

5 Now gently release your arms down towards the ground in slow motion, until your hands are resting softly on the cushions.

GENTLE SITTING TWIST

This gentle turning helps to maintain flexibility of the spine while releasing muscular tension in the upper back, neck and shoulders.

1 Remain seated in the same position as for SPREADING OUT and place your hands softly on your knees.

2 Release the base of your spine down towards the floor. Feel your spine lengthen from the waist up to your neck and the top of your head. Be aware of the rhythm of your breathing.

3 As if the movement is coming from the ground, very slowly turn your upper body towards the left, keeping your spine vertical.

4 Bring your right arm across your body and hold your right thigh on or just above the knee. Relax your left arm from the shoulder and touch the floor lightly behind you without leaning back, or put your hand behind your back if it does not reach the floor.

5 Let the turning movement continue upwards through your upper back and neck so that your head turns last of all to look over your left shoulder.

6 Breathe evenly and hold for three cycles of your normal rhythm, then come back slowly to the centre and repeat on the other side.

Remember

The turning movement should be slow and gentle, allowing time for your body to relax into the position as you breathe. Keep your spine vertical with your lower back releasing downwards throughout.

LEGS WIDE

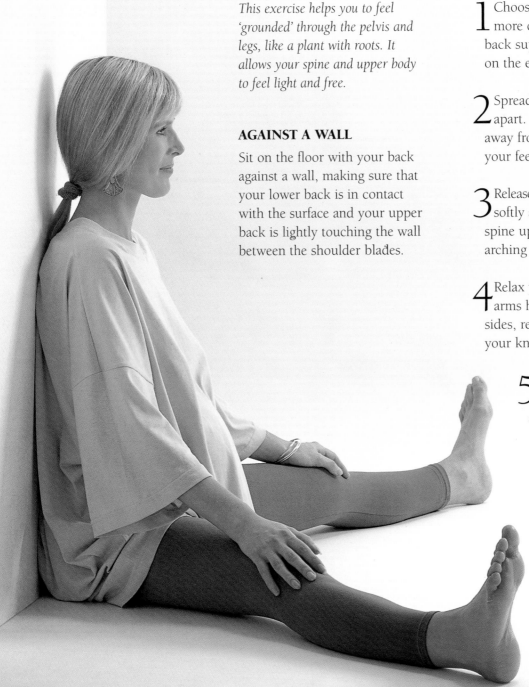

This exercise helps you to feel 'grounded' through the pelvis and legs, like a plant with roots. It allows your spine and upper body to feel light and free.

AGAINST A WALL

Sit on the floor with your back against a wall, making sure that your lower back is in contact with the surface and your upper back is lightly touching the wall between the shoulder blades.

1 Choose whichever position feels more comfortable, either with your back supported by a wall or sitting on the edge of a small cushion.

2 Spread your legs comfortably wide apart. Gently extend your heels away from your body and then relax your feet.

3 Release your lower back downwards softly and then gently lengthen your spine up towards your neck without arching in the back of the waist.

4 Relax your shoulders and let your arms hang down loosely by your sides, resting your hands softly on your knees.

5 Then, with your eyes open or closed, bring your awareness to your breathing.

> **Remember**
> Use this position every day. Avoid straining by opening your legs too wide – comfortably wide is good enough!

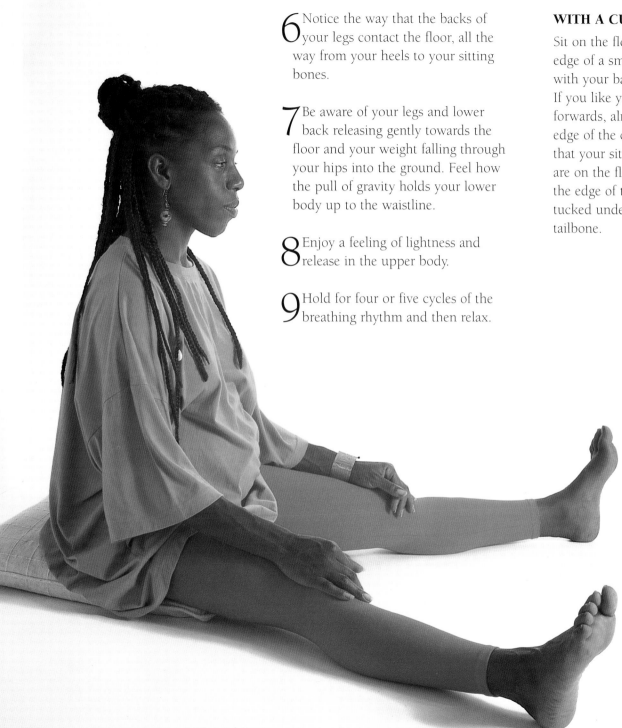

6 Notice the way that the backs of your legs contact the floor, all the way from your heels to your sitting bones.

7 Be aware of your legs and lower back releasing gently towards the floor and your weight falling through your hips into the ground. Feel how the pull of gravity holds your lower body up to the waistline.

8 Enjoy a feeling of lightness and release in the upper body.

9 Hold for four or five cycles of the breathing rhythm and then relax.

WITH A CUSHION

Sit on the floor on the edge of a small cushion with your back upright. If you like you can slide forwards, almost off the edge of the cushion, so that your sitting bones are on the floor, with the edge of the cushion tucked under your tailbone.

TAILOR POSITION

Tailor sitting is one of the most beneficial exercises for pregnancy. It encourages a feeling of openness in the pelvis and helps to release tension in the groin, while improving flexibility of the hip joints. Circulation to the pelvic area improves, and the pelvic floor muscles relax and release. The natural widening of the pelvis is gently encouraged, making it easier for your baby's head to engage in late pregnancy. If you suffer from back pain always practise tailor sitting with your lower back supported by a wall.

USING CUSHIONS

Tuck a cushion or two underneath each knee so that your legs are well supported.

1 Bend both knees and bring your feet together, placing them at a comfortable distance from your body.

2 Place the soles of your feet together so that the outside edges of the feet are touching.

3 Softly release your lower back downwards and then, keeping it down, gently lengthen your spine from the waist up towards the top of your head.

4 Relax and spread your shoulders and rest your hands comfortably on your legs.

5 Relax the back of your neck and your jaw, breathe evenly, and hold the position for up to five minutes.

6 Using your hands, bring your knees together gently to come out of the position.

WITHOUT CUSHIONS

You may prefer to do this exercise without cushions. However, if you do not feel completely comfortable like this, it is best to support the knees with cushions.

Remember

Keep your feet a little distance away from your body so that there is no feeling of strain in the groin. Avoid pushing or bouncing the knees. If you have pain in the pubic area, use extra cushions and place the feet farther forwards, or leave out this exercise.

LEGS WIDE LEANING BACK

Leaning back in either of these positions allows you to let go of your legs and relax your lower back. This encourages the release of tension in your legs and groin and the feeling of being grounded once you return to the upright position.

1 Sit in the LEGS WIDE position (page 24) with or without a cushion but away from the wall. Lean back slightly and support your upper body with your arms, placing your hands on the floor behind you.

2 Relax your shoulders and the back of your neck. Gently widen and open your chest so that your breathing can flow evenly. Release your lower back downwards towards the floor.

3 Now close your eyes for a moment or two and relax your legs completely, letting go of them to the ground.

4 Focus your awareness on your breathing rhythm and on the contact your body makes with the earth.

5 Remain in the position for four or five cycles of the breathing rhythm and then open your eyes and return slowly to sitting upright.

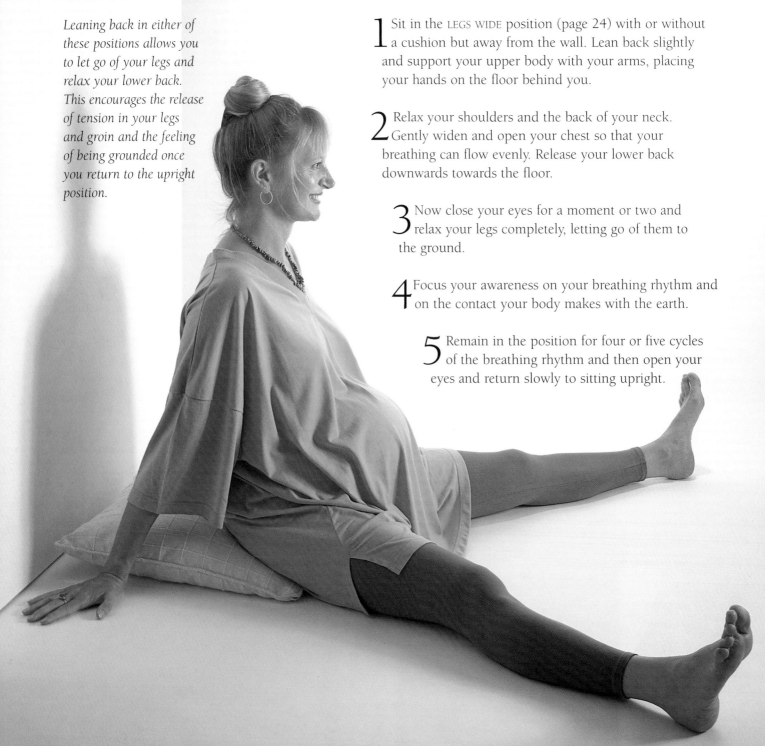

TAILOR SITTING LEANING BACK

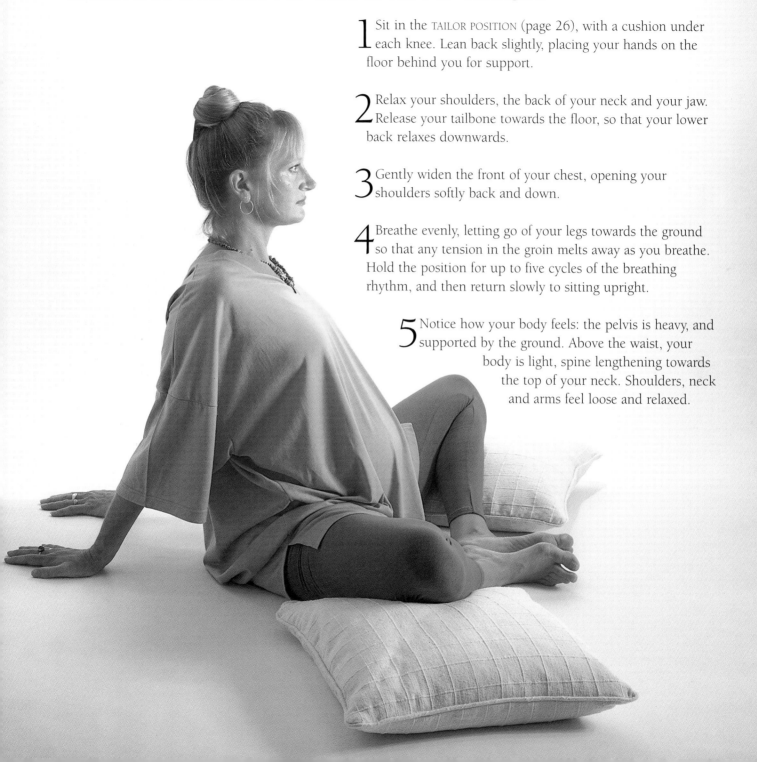

1 Sit in the TAILOR POSITION (page 26), with a cushion under each knee. Lean back slightly, placing your hands on the floor behind you for support.

2 Relax your shoulders, the back of your neck and your jaw. Release your tailbone towards the floor, so that your lower back relaxes downwards.

3 Gently widen the front of your chest, opening your shoulders softly back and down.

4 Breathe evenly, letting go of your legs towards the ground so that any tension in the groin melts away as you breathe. Hold the position for up to five cycles of the breathing rhythm, and then return slowly to sitting upright.

5 Notice how your body feels: the pelvis is heavy, and supported by the ground. Above the waist, your body is light, spine lengthening towards the top of your neck. Shoulders, neck and arms feel loose and relaxed.

SITTING WELL

This exercise can be done while you are working at a desk or eating a meal. By paying attention throughout the day to your posture while sitting, you can prevent strain in your lower back, keep your neck and shoulders relaxed and, in late pregnancy, help your baby to lie in a good position.

1 Sit on a chair or kneeling stool, making sure that it is comfortable and at the right height for the desk or table. You should be able to use your arms freely while keeping your shoulders relaxed and spine upright.

2 Feel the way your body weight falls through your sitting bones onto the seat, and softly release your lower back downwards, so that you feel securely 'grounded' in the pelvis.

3 Gently lengthen your spine from the back of your waist up towards the top of your head, without arching or pulling up in your lower back. Relax your tummy muscles.

4 Relax your shoulders opening wide across the front of the chest and releasing them back and down.

USING A KNEELING STOOL

Sit on the kneeling stool, placing your knees comfortably apart and relaxing your feet. Make sure that your weight is in your pelvis rather than resting on your knees, adjusting the height of the seat if necessary.

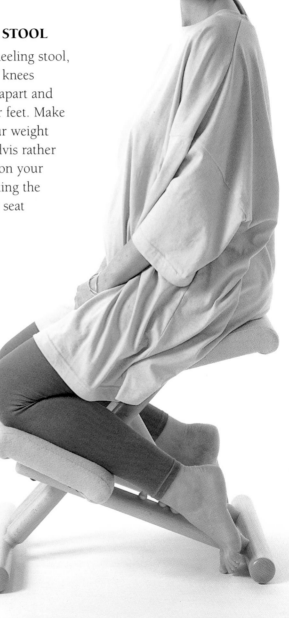

5 Raise your breast bone slightly to make space for your baby and relax your arms.

6 Relax the back of your neck and your jaw, allowing your head to find its balance, and breathe evenly in your normal rhythm.

SITTING ON A CHAIR

Choose a chair that allows you to sit with your feet flat on the floor so that your legs are relaxed. Place one or two cushions on the seat of the chair to raise your pelvis a little higher than your knees. Sit well back on the chair so that the base of your spine is supported by the back of the chair or use a cushion behind you to avoid leaning back.

Separate your knees and position your feet so that they can rest comfortably flat on the floor with heels down.

Avoid crossing your legs when sitting on a chair.

Remember

Avoid spending more than half an hour sitting at a stretch.

Get up and walk around for a few minutes if your work involves long hours at a desk. Close your eyes for a few moments every now and again and focus on the rhythm of your breathing and the presence of your baby.

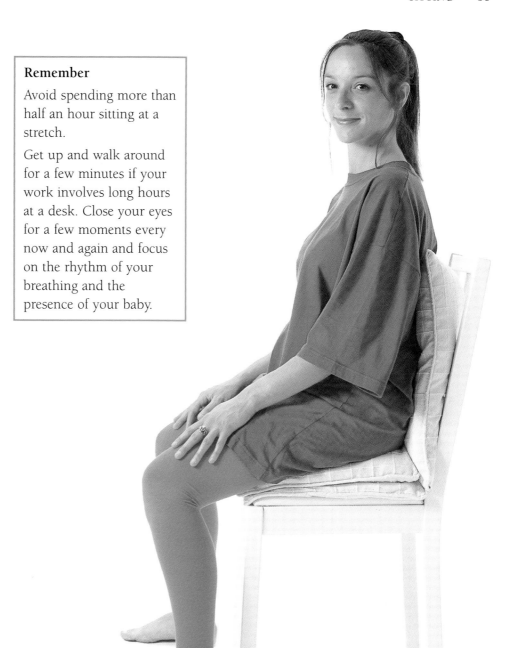

UPRIGHT CHILD'S POSE

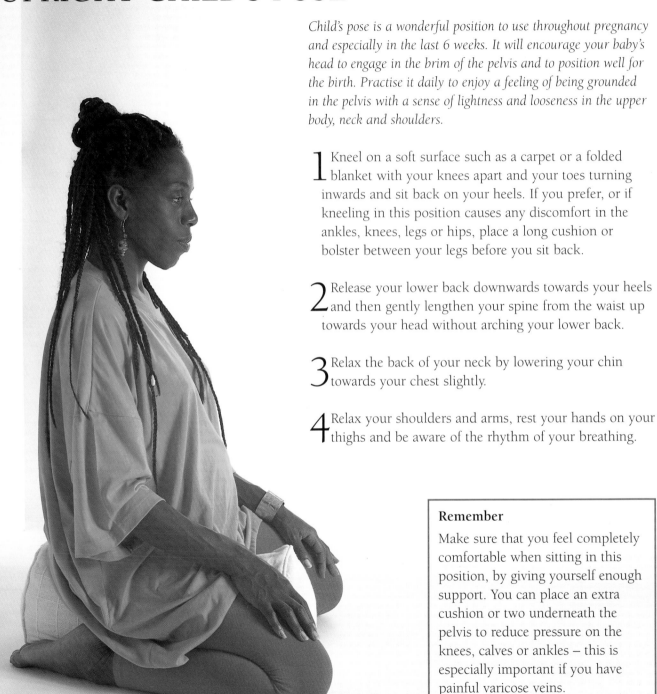

Child's pose is a wonderful position to use throughout pregnancy and especially in the last 6 weeks. It will encourage your baby's head to engage in the brim of the pelvis and to position well for the birth. Practise it daily to enjoy a feeling of being grounded in the pelvis with a sense of lightness and looseness in the upper body, neck and shoulders.

1 Kneel on a soft surface such as a carpet or a folded blanket with your knees apart and your toes turning inwards and sit back on your heels. If you prefer, or if kneeling in this position causes any discomfort in the ankles, knees, legs or hips, place a long cushion or bolster between your legs before you sit back.

2 Release your lower back downwards towards your heels and then gently lengthen your spine from the waist up towards your head without arching your lower back.

3 Relax the back of your neck by lowering your chin towards your chest slightly.

4 Relax your shoulders and arms, rest your hands on your thighs and be aware of the rhythm of your breathing.

Remember

Make sure that you feel completely comfortable when sitting in this position, by giving yourself enough support. You can place an extra cushion or two underneath the pelvis to reduce pressure on the knees, calves or ankles – this is especially important if you have painful varicose veins.

LENGTHENING

This exercise allows you to be aware of your spine lengthening in two directions at the same time – from the waist down towards the ground, and from the waist up towards the sky.

1 Start in the UPRIGHT CHILD'S POSE opposite with or without a long cushion or bolster. Focus your awareness on the heavy base of your spine. Be aware of your breathing.

2 Gently release your lower back downwards and, at the same time, begin slowly to raise your arms.

3 Allow your arms to come up over your head while keeping your awareness on releasing your lower back downwards.

4 Relax your shoulders downwards as your arms lengthen towards the sky. Keep your wrists soft and loose and hold the position for two to three cycles of the breath, breathing evenly.

5 With arms still raised, progress directly to LEANING FORWARDS (page 34), or lower your arms gently

---

Remember

Keep your weight centred in your pelvis and avoid arching in the back of your waist. Keep your arms and shoulders loose and relaxed with a gentle feeling of lengthening from the grounded base of the spine upwards; think of a plant growing towards the light from its roots in the earth.

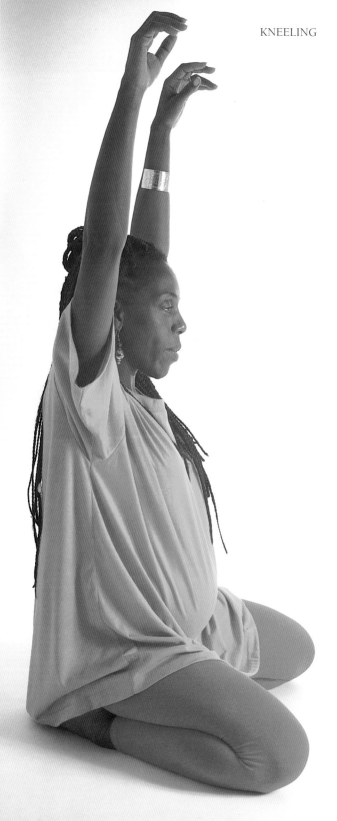

LEANING FORWARDS

This movement gently tips your pelvis forwards from the hips, taking the weight of your baby off your lower back. It encourages your baby to find a good position in the womb, while improving flexibility in your hips, knees and ankles.

Remember

Your spine should feel loose and relaxed and should not be bending – the forward movement comes from your hips. Your pelvis rests on your heels, or on the bolster if you are using one, throughout this exercise.

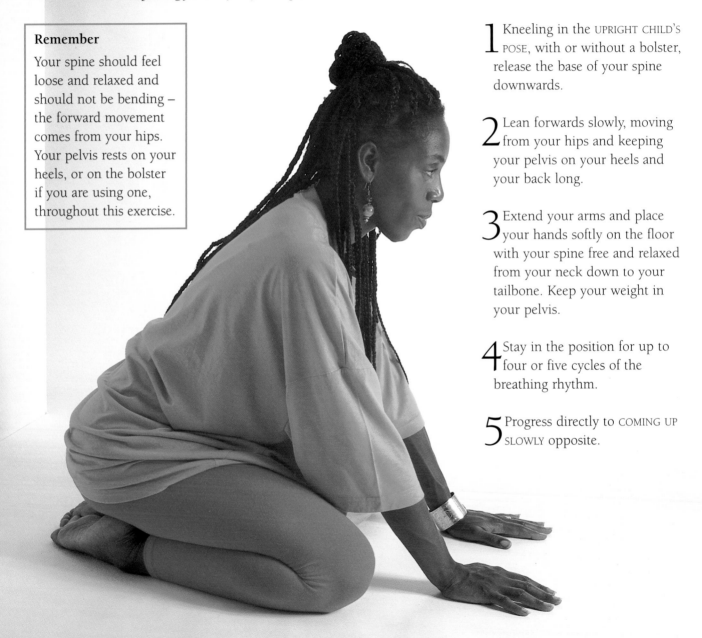

1 Kneeling in the UPRIGHT CHILD'S POSE, with or without a bolster, release the base of your spine downwards.

2 Lean forwards slowly, moving from your hips and keeping your pelvis on your heels and your back long.

3 Extend your arms and place your hands softly on the floor with your spine free and relaxed from your neck down to your tailbone. Keep your weight in your pelvis.

4 Stay in the position for up to four or five cycles of the breathing rhythm.

5 Progress directly to COMING UP SLOWLY opposite.

COMING UP SLOWLY

Use this exercise to return to UPRIGHT CHILD'S POSE *(page 32) whenever you come up from kneeling forwards. This will help you to keep your centre of gravity in the pelvis and protect your spine. Once you are upright you will enjoy a feeling of lightness in the upper body, neck and shoulders.*

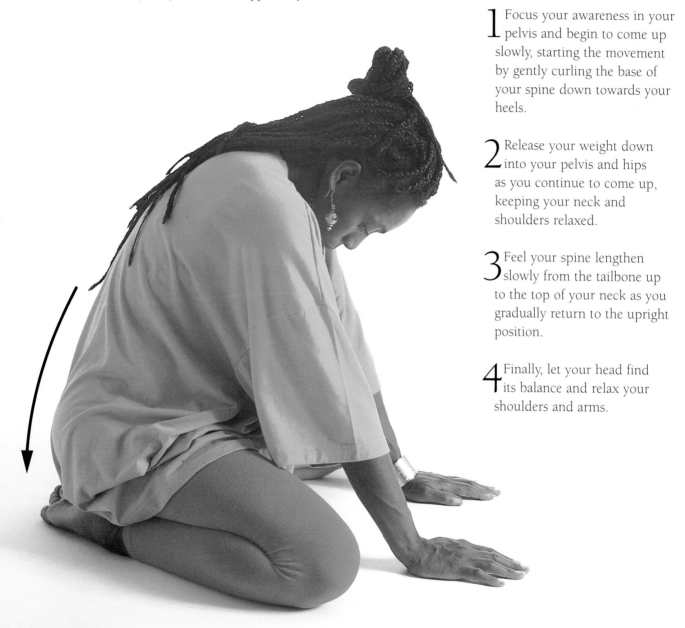

1 Focus your awareness in your pelvis and begin to come up slowly, starting the movement by gently curling the base of your spine down towards your heels.

2 Release your weight down into your pelvis and hips as you continue to come up, keeping your neck and shoulders relaxed.

3 Feel your spine lengthen slowly from the tailbone up to the top of your neck as you gradually return to the upright position.

4 Finally, let your head find its balance and relax your shoulders and arms.

RESTING OVER A BEANBAG

When you are in this position, the weight of your baby falls forwards, allowing your spine to relax completely, which can help to ease or prevent backache. Spending a little time every day in this position in late pregnancy helps your baby to find the best position for birth.

1 Place a large beanbag or a few large cushions in front of you on the floor. Kneel in UPRIGHT CHILD'S POSE (page 32), using a bolster between your legs if kneeling is uncomfortable, with the beanbag close to your knees.

2 Release the base of your spine downwards. Lean forwards slowly from your hips, keeping your pelvis on your heels. Relax onto the beanbag so that your upper body is completely supported and your spine feels free.

3 Make yourself comfortable, spreading your shoulders and placing your arms loosely on the beanbag. Rest your head with your neck in line with the rest of the spine.

4 Close your eyes and focus your awareness on the rhythm of your breathing, and on the heavy base of your spine. Spend about five minutes relaxing in this position.

5 Return to the upright position using steps 1–4 in COMING UP SLOWLY, page 35.

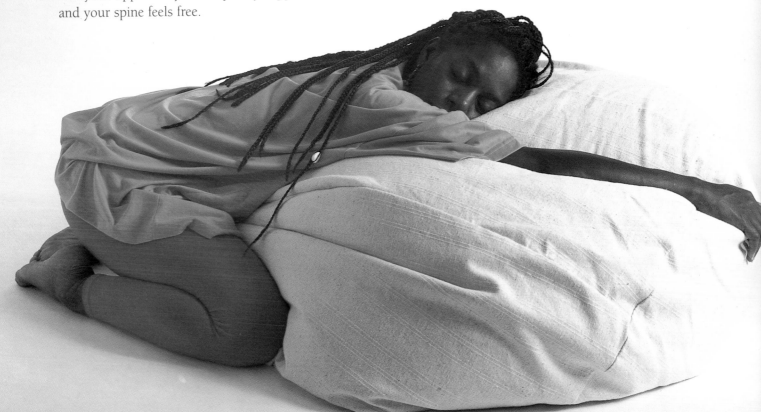

FORWARD STRETCH

If you find this movement easy and comfortable, you may enjoy this gentle stretch which helps to relax your lower back and release tension in the spine, shoulders and neck.

1 Kneel in UPRIGHT CHILD'S POSE (page 32) without a bolster. Release the base of your spine downwards and keep your pelvis on your heels throughout this exercise.

2 Release your upper body forwards slowly, moving from your hips and keeping your back straight and your spine free.

3 Progress farther forwards in easy stages, first onto your hands as in LEANING FORWARDS (page 34) and then onto your elbows.

4 Extend your arms out fully in front of you, placing your forehead on the ground or on a small cushion. Focus your awareness on the rhythm of your breathing and on the ground underneath your body.

5 Relax completely for up to a minute, breathing evenly, and then return to the upright position by COMING UP SLOWLY.

Remember

This exercise is not essential but is enjoyable if you find the movement easy. If your back bends or if you feel any strain or discomfort as you go forwards, leave it out, or do RESTING OVER A BEANBAG opposite instead.

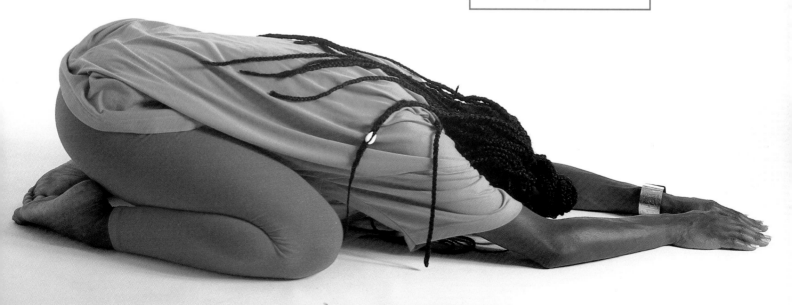

BABY HAMMOCK

This simple exercise releases tension in the lower back and prevents or eases backache. Kneeling on your hands and knees in late pregnancy encourages your baby's spine to rotate downwards towards the ground with the pull of gravity, allowing the baby's back to lie in the 'hammock' of your tummy muscles. This is called the 'anterior position' and is the best way your baby can lie for labour and birth. This exercise helps to prevent the baby lying 'posterior' (spine against your spine) as the birth approaches.

1 Kneel down and place your palms under your shoulders on the floor. If your wrists are swollen or aching, rest your hands on a soft pillow, or do this exercise leaning forwards onto the seat of a low chair with your arms folded and your back horizontal.

2 Put your knees in line with your hands and your feet in line with your knees.

3 Relax your neck and gently let go of the weight of your head. Breathe evenly and feel the way your hands and knees make contact with the floor.

**HANDS, FEET AND
KNEES IN LINE**

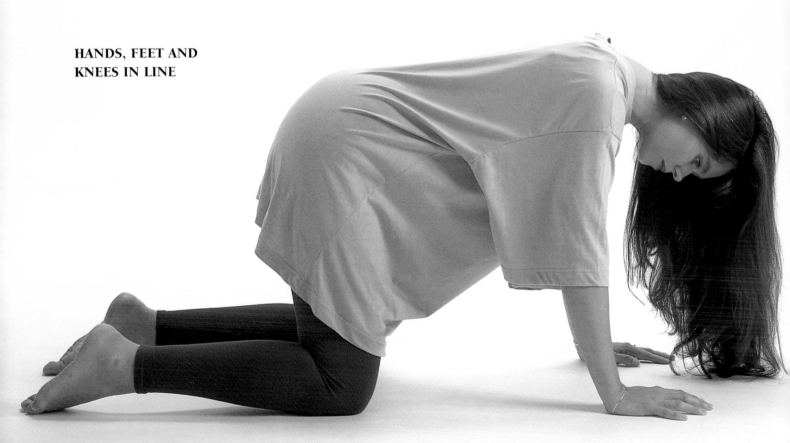

4 Breathe out slowly and lengthen the base of your spine gently downwards towards your heels so that your back becomes softly rounded like a bridge. Notice how your pelvis tucks under when your lower back lengthens downwards.

5 At the end of the out breath, gently tighten and squeeze your buttock muscles and hold for just a second or two, before returning to the starting position with your back horizontal as you inhale.

6 Repeat these movements up to ten times, moving gently with the wave of the breath.

Remember
Make these movements softly without tensing any muscles as your pelvis tucks under. Avoid arching or hollowing your lower back when you breathe in.

PELVIC TUCK

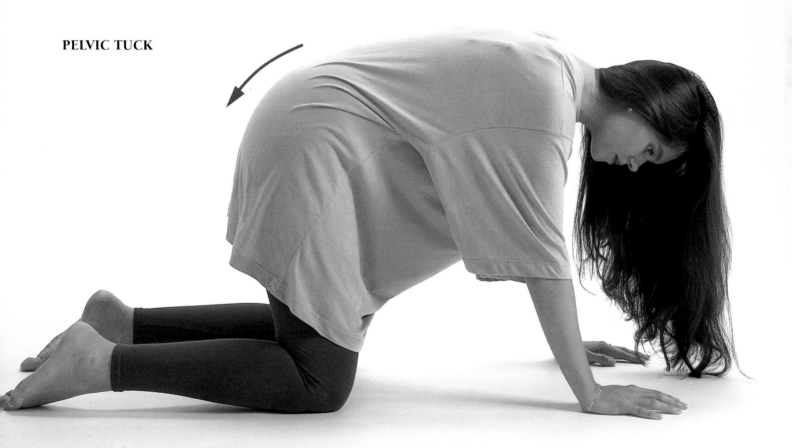

STANDING WELL

Good posture is especially important in pregnancy, when the extra weight you are carrying exaggerates the spinal curves. Any imbalance can cause back pain or sciatica. Lengthening your lower back downwards helps to prevent excess arching at the back of the waist – a common cause of back pain in pregnancy. Do this exercise daily, and remember it whenever you have to stand, for example, in a queue. If you feel faint when standing still for a few minutes, then leave out this exercise or remain in it very briefly for just a few seconds.

1 Stand with your feet about 30cm/12in (hips' width) apart. Position your feet so that they are parallel and then place your heels slightly wider apart than your toes.

2 Lift and spread all your toes and then relax them on the floor and repeat this twice more. Check that your knees are loose and relaxed so that the energy can flow through your legs.

3 Stroke down your lower back with your hands and, as you do so, gently release the heavy base of your spine downwards, as if you had a long, heavy tail.

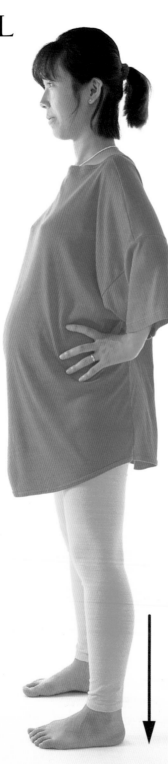

4 Place your hands on your hips for a few seconds, then relax and drop your shoulders, letting your arms hang loosely by your sides. Relax the back of your neck by releasing your chin down slightly towards your chest.

5 Breathe evenly and sense how your body is attracted to the earth from the pelvis down, and to the sky from the waist up. Feel how your body weight drops down through your lower back towards the ground through your hips, legs and feet.

6 Hold for a few cycles of the breathing rhythm, moving out of the position whenever you want to.

Remember
Always keep your heels slightly wider apart than your toes and your lower back releasing downwards when you stand and walk. This may feel strange, or 'pigeon-toed', at first but once you get used to it, you will sense how widening your heels releases tension in your lower back, spine and shoulders.

BENDING FORWARDS

This movement allows you to release tension in the back of your legs, to lengthen and release your spine and relax your shoulders at the same time. Try doing it at the kitchen counter or table while you are waiting for the kettle to boil! However, do not do this exercise if bending forward makes you feel light-headed.

1 Face a table or counter in the STANDING WELL start position opposite. Release your lower back downwards and drop your weight through your heels into the floor. Breathe evenly.

2 Keep dropping your heels and breathe out as you slowly lower your upper body forwards, bending from your hips. Place your palms on the table top with arms outstretched.

3 Be aware of the heavy base of your spine, and lengthen and release the rest of the spine from the waistline towards the top of your neck.

4 Hold the position for a few seconds, enjoying a feeling of relaxation and release along the spine and a gentle stretch at the back of your legs. Be aware of the pull of gravity through your heels now and also when coming up.

Remember
Your hips remain in line with your heels when you bend forwards. Your spine feels long and free and you feel the stretch in the back of your legs.

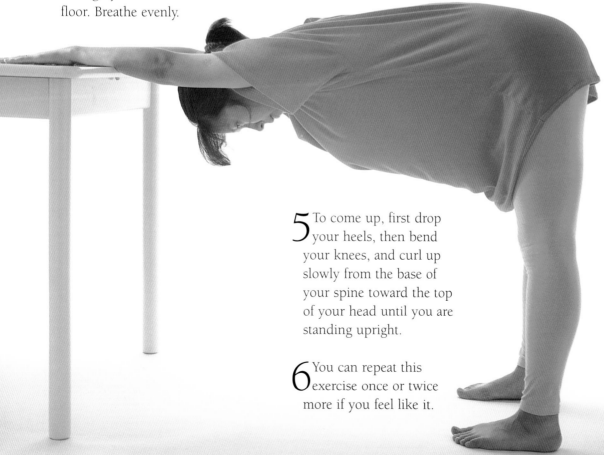

5 To come up, first drop your heels, then bend your knees, and curl up slowly from the base of your spine toward the top of your head until you are standing upright.

6 You can repeat this exercise once or twice more if you feel like it.

GENTLE STANDING TWIST

For releasing tension in the back, neck and shoulders, and maintaining flexibility of the spine.

1 Place a stool in front of you. Stand in position as for STANDING WELL start (page 40) with your lower back releasing towards the floor, and your arms and shoulders relaxed. Breathe evenly and feel the contact your feet make with the floor as your weight settles into your heels.

2 Place your left foot on the stool in front of you, making sure that your feet are still parallel. Breathe and slowly turn your upper body to the left, keeping your feet and hips facing forwards. As your spine gently turns from the base up to the top of your neck, relax both shoulders and take your right arm across your body, holding softly the far side of your bent knee.

3 Let your left arm hang loosely from the shoulder as your head and neck turn gently to the left. Release the left shoulder down and back and hold the position for about three to five cycles of the breathing rhythm. Slowly come back to facing forwards.

4 With both feet still in position, turn your body to the right, taking your right hand over your knee and holding gently on the other side of your thigh.

5 Look round over your right shoulder, relaxing the arm and releasing the shoulder softly back and down. Hold for three to five cycles of the breathing rythm and then come slowly back to facing forwards. Return to the standing position.

6 Repeat the exercise, placing your right foot on the stool, turning first to the right, and then to the left. Return to the basic standing position.

Remember
Turn gently without straining. Feel the contact the foot of your straight leg is making with the ground as the weight falls through the heel.

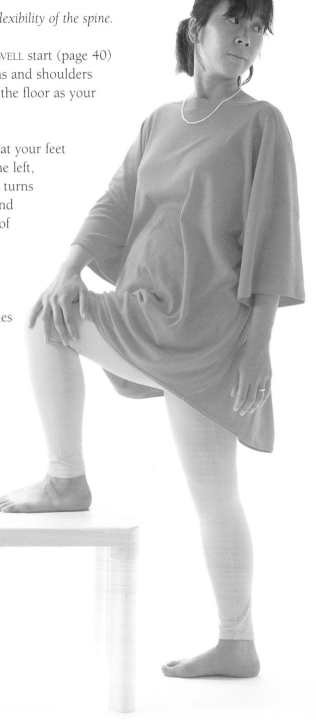

CALF STRETCH

This exercise lengthens and relaxes the calf and hamstring muscles at the back of the legs. Regular practice will help to relieve leg cramps and will also improve your squatting.

1 Stand about 30cm/12in away from a wall with your feet parallel. Clasp your hands and place your forearms on the wall, relaxing your neck and shoulders.

2 Take your left leg back and your right leg forwards with the left knee straight and the right knee bending. Check that your feet are parallel and facing the wall and your hips are in line, parallel to the wall, with your shoulders relaxed.

3 Breathe evenly and drop the back heel onto the floor, opening the back of the knee. Your front foot rests lightly on the ground while your weight falls through into your back heel. Feel the stretch in the back of your left leg and hold the position, breathing evenly for three to five cycles of the breathing rhythm.

4 Change legs so that the left leg is forward with the knee bent and the right leg back. Breathe evenly and hold the position for three to five cycles of the breath and then change legs. Repeat the exercise once more on both legs and then return to STANDING WELL (page 40).

SQUATTING
USING A STOOL

Squatting in pregnancy helps improve flexibility of the pelvic joints and gently increase the pelvic diameters. Squatting on a stool like this will encourage your baby's head to engage in late pregnancy. Use this position in preference to a full squat in the last six weeks of pregnancy or if you find squatting difficult.

1 Put a small cushion on a low stool or pile of heavy books about 25cm/10in high, and position it against a wall. Stand with your feet a little wider apart than in the STANDING WELL position (page 40) and slightly turn them out.

2 Feel the way your feet contact the floor and breathe evenly, releasing your weight down through your heels into the ground.

3 On an out breath, bend your knees a little, keeping your heels down on the ground.

4 Slowly continue this movement until your pelvis drops down gently into a squatting position, with your sitting bones resting on the stool and your knees wide apart in line with your feet.

5 Relax and lengthen your spine against the surface of the wall.

6 Remain in this position for up to five minutes and then come up slowly.

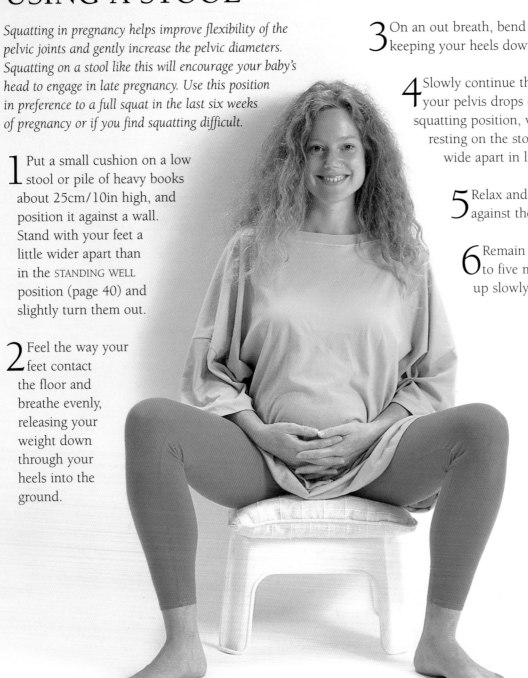

> **Remember**
> Squatting on a stool reduces pressure on the cervix and pelvic floor. In the last six weeks of pregnancy, or if you have haemorrhoids, vulval varicosities, full or partial placenta praevia or a cervical suture, squat in this position only and avoid the positions shown on pages 45–47.

HOLDING ON

This supported squat is slightly more challenging than the previous one and can be practised up to 34 weeks of pregnancy. If you find it too difficult or uncomfortable, stick to using a stool. Otherwise, it is a good idea to alternate using a stool and holding on when you practise.

1 Stand facing a firm support, such as the edge of a table, a window ledge or the side of the bath. Place your feet apart as in the previous exercise and breathe evenly, dropping your weight into the floor through your heels.

2 Hold on to the support and, keeping your heels down throughout and your arms straight, bend your knees and slowly lower your pelvis into a squat. Your knees should be spread comfortably wide apart, with your feet following the angle of your knees.

3 Breathe evenly and hold the position for about three cycles of the breathing rhythm.

4 Drop your heels and come up slowly on an out breath.

5 Repeat this exercise two or three times.

Remember
Keep your spine nice and long and avoid bending your back when you squat.

Do not do this exercise in the last 6 weeks of pregnancy.

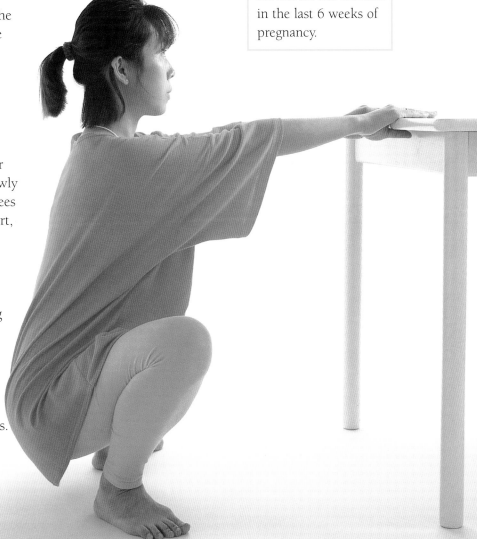

FULL SQUAT

Do this exercise only if you feel completely at ease USING A STOOL *or* HOLDING ON *(pages 44–45). It can be practised up to 34 weeks of pregnancy. Support under the heels makes squatting easier for some people, but if you are not completely comfortable then leave out this exercise.*

USING A ROLL

Roll up an exercise mat or a thin blanket and put it on the floor. Stand with your feet apart as in USING A STOOL (page 44), only this time place the roll under your heels and stand with your feet apart and slightly turned out.

1 Come down slowly into a squat, bending your knees and lowering your pelvis as your weight falls through the heels into the floor.

2 Clasp your hands and place your elbows inside your knees, spreading your knees comfortably apart with your feet following the angle of your knees. Avoid turning your feet out too much.

3 Lengthen your spine, leaning forwards slightly from your hips if it feels comfortable.

4 Breathe evenly and hold for three to five cycles of the breath.

5 Come up slowly, dropping your weight into your heels, or roll forwards on your hands and knees and then come up.

WITHOUT SUPPORT

Stand as before with your feet apart and slightly turned out. Drop your heels and breathe evenly. Use this position only if you find it easy to achieve and completely comfortable.

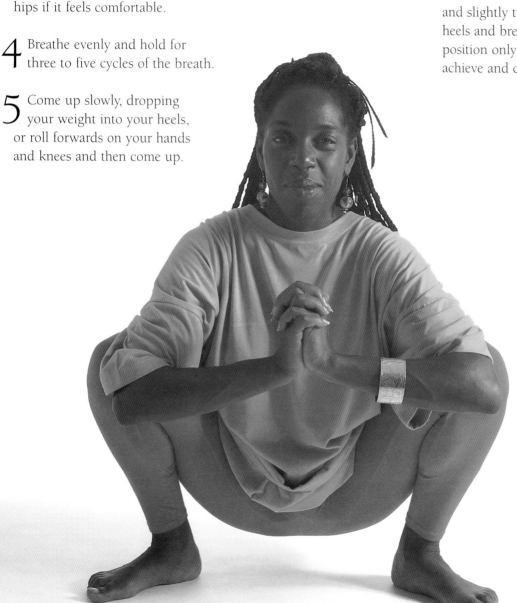

Remember

Keep your spine long and avoid bending your back. In the last 6 weeks of pregnancy it is best to use a stool and to keep your spine upright against a wall when you squat (page 44). This will help your baby's head to engage.

THE PELVIC FLOOR

Strengthening your pelvic floor will help you in pregnancy and during and after the birth. There are two special exercises which you can practise regularly while you are pregnant, called QUICKIES (pages 50–51) and THE LIFT (pages 52–53), and four positions in which you can do them. Before you try them out you should understand where your pelvic floor is, how it functions and why these exercises are so important.

What is the pelvic floor ?

Inside the base of your bony pelvis there is a layer of muscle shaped rather like a hammock which forms the floor of your pelvis. It extends across the outlet of your pelvis, from your pubic bone in front to your tailbone at the back, and also from side to side, from one sitting bone to the other. The muscle fibres of the pelvic floor are arranged in three inter-connecting rings or 'sphincters' surrounding the openings to the pelvic organs: in front, the urethra (leading to the bladder); in the centre, the vagina (leading to the uterus); and at the back, the anus (leading to the bowel).

The function of the pelvic floor

The pelvic floor supports the weight of your pelvic and abdominal organs, including your uterus, and the weight of your baby while you are pregnant. The muscles also control the opening and closing of your bladder and bowel. Your

baby's head and body will pass through the centre of the pelvic floor when you give birth. The muscle fibres soften and relax in pregnancy to allow this to happen more easily. Then after the birth they regain their strength and tone.

The benefits of exercising the pelvic floor

Pelvic floor exercises involve both tightening and contracting movements as well as releasing and letting go and have two important benefits:
1 The tightening or contracting movements improve muscle tone and strengthen the pelvic floor. This ensures that there is good support for the increasing weight of the pelvic and abdominal organs in pregnancy. Good muscle tone will also maintain control of the opening and closing of the bladder and bowel and improve or prevent problems such as incontinence, vulval varicosities and piles (haemorrhoids). These problems arise when the muscle tone of the pelvic floor is too slack. They are more common in pregnancy, when these muscles become softer in readiness for the birth. Doing pelvic floor exercises regularly while you are pregnant lessens the risk of damage to the pelvic floor during childbirth and also results in good muscle tone and a quick recovery after the birth.
2 The relaxing and releasing movements help to prevent or ease constipation. Learning to focus your awareness on letting go of tension in the

pelvic floor, as you do when you release your pelvic floor muscles, also prepares you for giving birth when you will instinctively release and relax these muscles as your baby's head and body emerge.

How to tell whether you are using the right muscles

1 Next time you empty your bladder try stopping the flow in midstream. The muscles you will be contracting are your pelvic floor muscles. Now try tightening the same muscles after your bladder has emptied.

2 When you are in the bath, insert one finger in your vagina and tighten the muscles inside to grip your finger. These are your pelvic floor muscles. When you tighten or contract these muscles you will find that the front, centre and back of your pelvic floor all move in unison.

Don't worry if, at first, your buttock or stomach muscles move as well – with practice you will learn to move your pelvic floor muscles on their own.

Positions for pelvic floor exercises

Pelvic floor exercises can be done in four different positions – **all fours**, **knee chest**, **half squat** and **easy squat** – shown below and on pages 50–53. You can choose any one of them for both exercises and vary your choice each time you practise or change your position midway.

If you have piles (haemorrhoids) or vulval varicosities in pregnancy, regular practice of these exercises will help to improve or eliminate discomfort. However, do them only in the **all fours** or **knee chest** positions on pages 50–51 and omit the squatting positions.

How often should I do pelvic floor exercises?

Once you have chosen the position you want and are comfortable, do both THE LIFT and QUICKIES in sucession. Try to do this during your exercise session at least three times a week. QUICKIES can be done on their own at any time and in any place, as often as you like, but once a day is plenty!

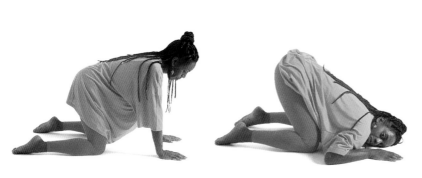

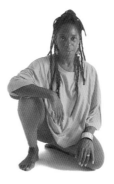

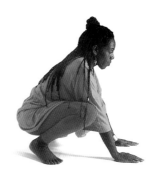

All fours   Knee chest   Half squat   Easy squat

QUICKIES

Quickies encourage good muscle tone of the pelvic floor and are easy to do on a daily basis. Do them in any of the positions shown on pages 50–53. You can go on doing these after giving birth to strengthen your pelvic floor and aid your recovery postnatally.

1 Choose one of the four positions and make yourself comfortable, breathing in your normal rhythm.

2 Focus your awareness on your pelvic floor and tighten the muscles, pulling them up inside.

ALL FOURS

Kneel on your hands and knees, placing them about 30cm/12in apart, with your back flat like a table. Spread your palms and your fingers and make sure your feet are in line with your knees. Lower your head and relax your neck and shoulders. Feel the ground underneath you and breathe comfortably.

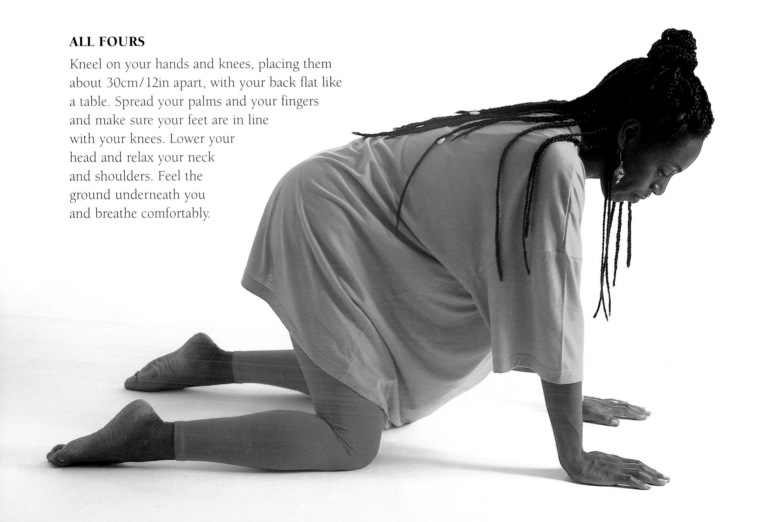

3 Hold to the count of five and then let go slowly.

4 Repeat the first two steps ten times and then stop.

5 Relax for a few moments and then repeat this exercise twice more.

KNEE CHEST

Start in the all fours position opposite. Lean forwards from your hips and place your lower arms on the ground. Turn your head and rest your face on the ground and relax your neck and shoulders. Focus on the ground underneath you and the flow of your breathing.

Remember

To relieve the discomfort of piles or vulval varicosities, try doing 50–100 quickies in the knee chest position first thing every morning and last thing every night. Keep it up every day until there is a definite improvement, and then continue to do 25–50 quickies twice every day in the knee chest position.

THE LIFT

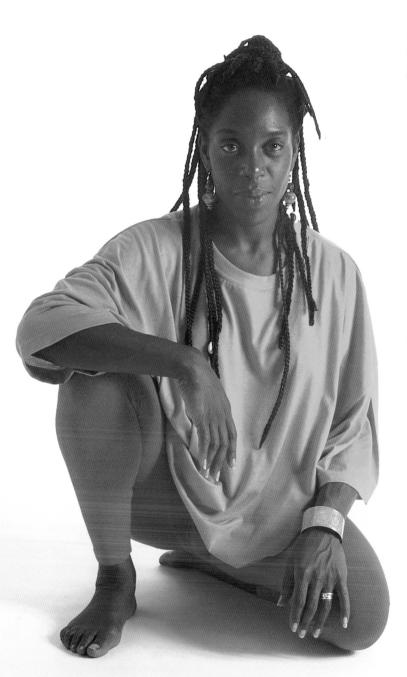

To help feel the pelvic muscles tightening little by little, imagine a lift in a four-storey building as you are doing this exercise. You will begin in the basement and then go up to the third floor. Pause briefly at each level on the way up and as you go back down again.

1 Make yourself comfortable in one of the four positions, breathing in your normal rhythm.

2 Close your eyes and focus awareness on your pelvic floor.

3 Start in the 'basement' and contract or tighten your pelvic floor muscles, drawing them up a little way towards your uterus and pausing on the 'ground floor'.

4 Now tighten a little more up to the 'first floor' and pause, up to the 'second floor' and pause, and then up to the third floor.

HALF SQUAT

Start by kneeling on the floor and sitting back on your heels, then bend one leg and place the foot flat on the floor. Position your arms and legs comfortably and relax your neck and shoulders. Be aware of the ground underneath you and the rhythm of your breathing.

5 Breathe normally while you hold the pelvic floor muscles tight on the top floor for a second or two.

6 Now gently release your pelvic floor muscles in stages as you descend, floor by floor. Pause at each level for a second on the way down.

7 Relax the pelvic floor completely as you descend to the basement, rest for a moment, and repeat the exercise twice.

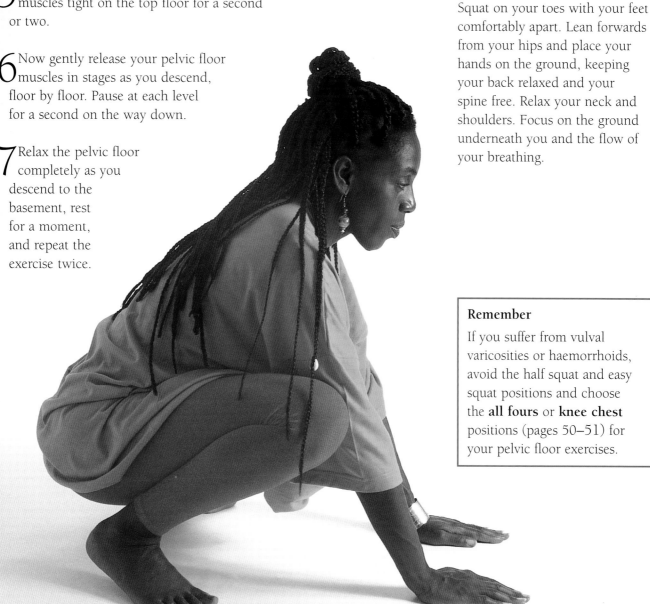

EASY SQUAT

Squat on your toes with your feet comfortably apart. Lean forwards from your hips and place your hands on the ground, keeping your back relaxed and your spine free. Relax your neck and shoulders. Focus on the ground underneath you and the flow of your breathing.

Remember

If you suffer from vulval varicosities or haemorrhoids, avoid the half squat and easy squat positions and choose the **all fours** or **knee chest** positions (pages 50–51) for your pelvic floor exercises.

PREPARATION FOR LABOUR

It is a good idea to prepare for labour throughout your pregnancy. If you practise the movements on page 57–61 they will soon become comfortable and familiar body habits and it will be easy and natural to use them later on in labour. You will also be encouraging your baby into a good position for the birth and helping your baby's head to 'engage' in the rim of your pelvis.

The last weeks of your pregnancy are special. You need to rest more and focus on preparing mentally and physically for your birth. This will enable you to approach the experience well rested and relaxed. Try to spend time, ideally an hour or so a day, doing your favourite exercises including BREATHING and BABY AWARENESS (pages 12–13), the RELAXATION positions on pages 62–65 and the exercises in this section.

Going into labour

Labour will start when your pregnancy reaches full term and your baby is ready to be born. This can happen any time between the 37th and 43rd week of pregnancy although the average length of pregnancy is 40–41 weeks. You may experience a 'pre-labour' in which mild contractions may last several hours or even overnight and then stop. This is very common and is getting your body ready for labour itself. The exercises you have been doing so far have been preparing you to

work through the contractions you will experience as labour becomes established. You have already been learning how to focus awareness on your breathing, how to be in contact with the ground underneath you, and how to relax your body and release tension while you exercise. This is all great practice for staying relaxed during your labour and for coping with the power and intensity of the contractions. After a while you will get used to the rhythm of working though the contractions and resting in between them. Usually pain builds up towards the peak of each contraction and gradually fades away by the end. The resting phases between contractions are pain free and give you a chance to relax and replenish your energy. It is a continual rhythm of work and rest, allowing your body to surrender as your uterus slowly opens to allow your baby to be born.

While the contractions themselves are intense and are likely to be painful at the peak, the peaceful rests in between make it possible to go along with this rhythmic process. A contraction lasts about 30 seconds in early labour, building up to a minute or one-and-a-half minutes by the time you are almost ready to give birth.

Think of your labour positively, as a personal birth dance. You are helping your baby to be born. Express yourself freely with your body and with movements to the pain, exploring which movements make you most comfortable. They will also be the best movements to help your baby on his or her way through the birth canal.

On the following pages you will find some easy upright movements and positions which you may find helpful to use when you are in labour.

Upright positions
Very few women, left to their own instincts, would choose to lie on their backs or in a semi-reclining position in labour. This is a custom which has developed in the Western world along with a more medical approach to birth. However, today it is being widely recognized that when mothers can move freely in labour and choose their own positions there are many benefits to both mother and baby. These include:
- More comfortable upright positions that reduce pain, helping you to be more in control of your labour.
- More effective contractions, so labour tends to be shorter.
- Improved blood supply to the baby, so there is less risk of foetal distress in labour.
- Easier journey for the baby through the pelvis, because the pelvic diameters are wider in upright positions and the downward force of gravity helps the baby to descend.

Using upright positions increases your chances of an uncomplicated birth and makes it less likely that you will need interventions. However, if you do need help or choose some medication, you will probably find that something you have learnt from your exercises will help you. You can approach the experience from a position of power and feel good about it in the end, as well as make a rapid recovery afterwards.

How to practise for labour
You will need a chair, a pillow, a low stool and a beanbag or a pile of large cushions for the exercises on pages 57–61. When you practise these movements, try to imagine that you are experiencing a real contraction in labour using a combination of position, movement and breathing to get through it. Think of the contraction like a wave in the ocean. It begins gently and gradually builds up in intensity to reach a peak, then it begins to ebb and decline until it's gone.

Choose one of the positions, then move your body freely in the position and focus at the same time on your breathing. Practise breathing your way over or through the wave of the contraction, concentrating on breathing out through your mouth and then inhaling slowly through your nose. There will be three to five cycles of the breathing rhythm per contraction.

Start as soon as the imaginary contraction begins, focusing on the out breaths and 'breathing pain away' through the peak of the contraction until it subsides. Then rest and relax for a while, using one of the resting positions suggested at the end of each exercise. Let go of your body and your mind completely when you are resting so that every muscle is relaxed. Breathe in your normal rhythm, in and out through your nose while resting. As the contractions get stronger you may find that you need to make more noise as you are breathing out. This will help you to release and let go of the pain. Step 3 of 'Breathing awareness for labour' (see next column) includes some breathing with sounds to help you prepare for this. Also, be aware of the earth underneath you and stay 'grounded' while in the midst of a contraction (see step 2).

In the weeks approaching birth, practise for labour every day for just five–ten minutes combining position, movements and breathing. On the day your labour happens for real, wait as long as possible until you are in established labour before you use the labour positions. When the contractions become so strong that you have to focus on them – that's when you begin to work with these positions.

There are three simple breathing exercises you can try in each of the labour positions shown on pages 57–61, moving your body freely as you imagine breathing through a contraction in labour. Afterwards, choose one of the recommended resting positions.

Breathing awareness for labour

1 Exhale slowly through your mouth so that you can hear the sound of the out breath. Pause at the end of each exhalation and inhale slowly through your nose. Continue for three to five cycles of the breathing rythm, and then relax in a resting position.

2 Repeat step 1 but focus your awareness on the contact your body is making with the ground. Direct the exhalations downwards as if to breathe the pain away into the earth each time you breathe out, and then breathe in slowly. Again, continue for three to five cycles of the breathing rhythm, and relax.

3 This time, repeat step 2 but try making some low vowel sounds as you exhale. Try ooooooh and aaaaah, releasing the sound from deep inside. Many women find that expressing sounds freely in labour helps to reduce pain. Continue with three to five cycles of the breathing rhythm, and relax.

STANDING

Standing up and moving during contractions helps to encourage the progress of labour. Leaning forwards as you move will ease the pain and position your baby positively. Relax in a resting position in between contractions (see below).

1 Stand with your feet well grounded and comfortably apart so that your whole body feels loose and relaxed.

2 Hold onto the back of a chair and bend your knees, rolling your hips slowly, making easy circular movements, or swing your hips slowly from side to side.

3 Work through a practise 'contraction' using the BREATHING AWARENESS exercises opposite, and then relax in a resting position.

RESTING POSITIONS

– Sit on a chair, knees apart and lean forwards, resting your upper body on a support (page 62).

– Sit astride the chair, facing backwards, resting on a pillow over the back of the chair.

– Do some easy supported squatting on a stool (page 44).

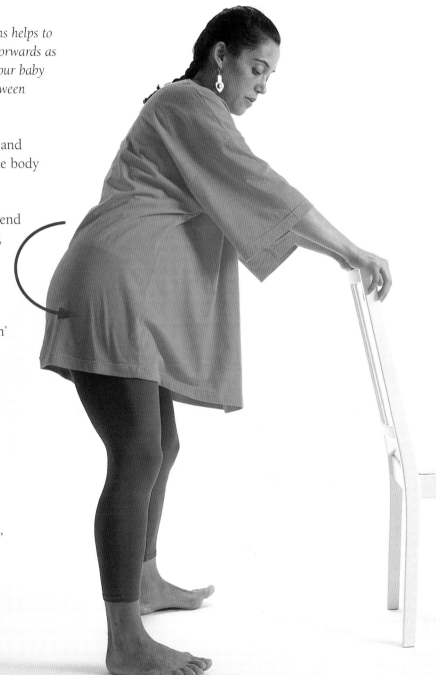

KNEELING UPRIGHT

*In this vertical kneeling position gravity will help
to make your contractions more effective. Use it
in labour if you still have quite a long way to go,
as an alternative to standing. This position can
also be used in a birth pool.*

1 Kneel on the floor on a soft surface with your
knees slightly apart. Relax your arms and
shoulders and rest your hands on your hips,
let them hang loosely by your sides or hold on
to a support.

2 Roll your hips, making soft, circular
movements, or alternatively swing your
hips from side to side.

3 Breathe through a few practice contractions,
using the BREATHING AWARENESS exercises on
page 56, and then relax in a resting position.

RESTING POSITIONS

– Lean forwards onto a pillow placed on the seat
  of a chair.
– Relax over a beanbag so that your upper body
  is completely supported (see page 63).

> **Remember**
> You may spend a long
> time kneeling in labour,
> so protect your knees by
> kneeling on some soft
> pillows or a foam mat.

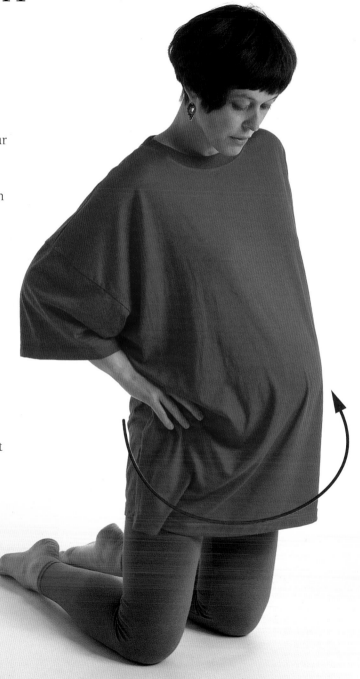

HALF KNEEL/HALF SQUAT

It may be helpful to use this as a variation on the kneeling positions from time to time during labour. Many women enjoy this position and find that it helps to relieve pain.

1 Begin in the kneeling upright position opposite on a soft surface to protect your knees. Lift one leg with the knee bent and foot on the floor.

2 Relax your shoulders and arms, placing your hands softly on your bent knee.

3 Breathing out, lunge gently forwards towards the bent knee.

4 Breathing in, come back slowly to the more upright starting position.

5 Repeat this movement four to five times and then change legs and repeat on the other side. Then relax in a resting position.

RESTING POSITIONS

– Kneel forwards onto a beanbag (see page 63).

– Squat supported on a stool, leaning forwards.

KNEELING ON ALL FOURS

Kneeling on all fours is a very secure position, offering you more support from the ground and a feeling of privacy, helping you to avoid distractions and focus on the contractions. This more horizontal kneeling will help you to stay in control during the very fast and intense contractions that occur towards the end of your labour. This is a useful position if you have a 'backache labour' and will encourage a baby in the posterior position to turn into the more favourable anterior position by the time you are ready to give birth.

1 Kneel on a soft surface on the ground, placing your palms down in line with your knees. You can increase your comfort during labour by placing a small cushion under each ankle.

2 Relax your neck and shoulders, letting go of the weight of your head. Breathe evenly and feel the way your hands and knees contact the floor.

3 Roll your hips, making soft circular movements, or swing your hips from side to side.

4 Work through the BREATHING AWARENESS exercises on page 56 while moving in this position, and then relax.

RESTING POSITION

From the kneeling position, lean forwards onto a beanbag or a pile of large cushions (see page 63) so that your whole body is supported.

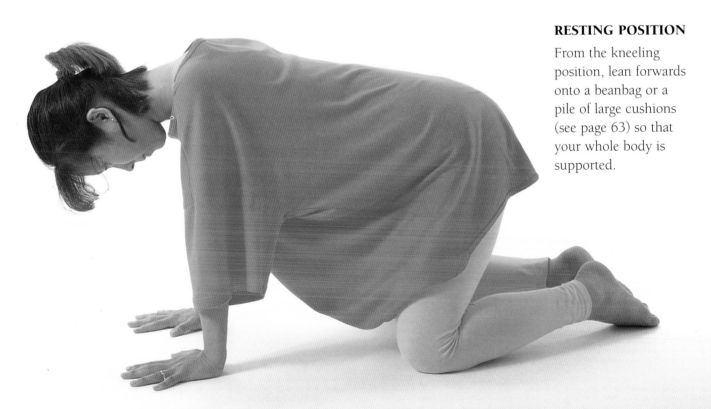

ROCKING

When kneeling on all fours in labour, it can be helpful to rock your body forwards and back and push into the ground with your hands as a gentle form of resistance. Move slowly and avoid arching your lower back when you come forwards.

1 Kneel on a soft surface on the floor on your hands and knees, with your knees comfortably apart. Focus your awareness on your breathing and on the contact your body is making with the ground.

2 On breathing in, bring your weight forwards onto your hands without arching your back.

3 Breathe out and bring your pelvis back towards your heels.

4 Repeat these movements five or six times, coming forwards on the in breath and back on the out breath, and then relax in the resting position.

5 Now try these movements using the BREATHING AWARENESS exercises on page 56.

RESTING POSITION

Kneel forwards over a beanbag (see page 63) or onto a support.

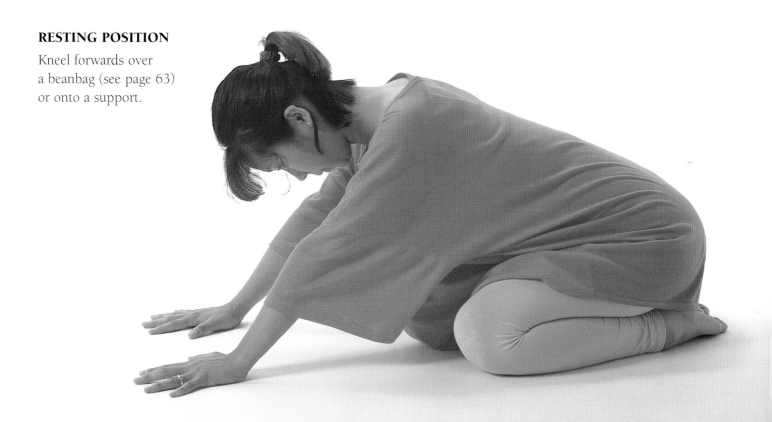

RELAXATION
AT A DESK

Your body is working hard while you are pregnant to provide nourishment for your growing baby and also to sustain and carry the increasing weight. Relaxation is very important and you will need to rest several times a day to avoid tiredness. Choose any one of the positions on pages 62–65 and remain in it for five minutes or longer, depending on how much spare time you have. Use this position to rest while you are working at a desk.

1 Sit on a chair with your knees comfortably wide apart and your feet flat on the floor with a cushion or support under your feet if necessary.

2 Lean forwards from your hips onto a table or desk with your head resting on your folded arms, or on a cushion or pillow.

3 Relax your neck and shoulders, release your lower back towards the chair and breathe evenly.

Remember
Five to ten minutes of relaxation is very helpful during a busy day. If you can, try to arrange to have a rest for at least half an hour after lunch.

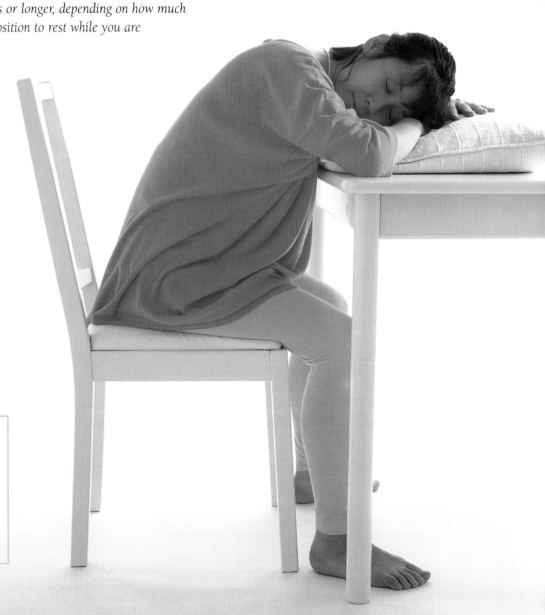

OVER A BEANBAG

This is a wonderful resting position as it takes the weight of your baby forwards, away from your lower back.
It helps to position your baby well for birth, and can be used for massage and also as a resting position in labour.

1 Kneel on a soft surface on the floor with your knees apart facing a beanbag. You can place an extra cushion or two between your buttocks and your calves for comfort.

2 Come forwards slowly from your hips, keeping your pelvis down on your heels, until your upper body can relax onto a beanbag or several big cushions.

3 Make yourself very comfortable, moulding the beanbag to fit your body, until you feel totally supported.

4 Spread your shoulders wide and rest your head, relaxing your arms on the beanbag.

Remember
If you feel any discomfort in your knees, calves or ankles, place cushions under your buttocks to raise your pelvis higher than your knees or kneel with a bolster cushion between your legs.

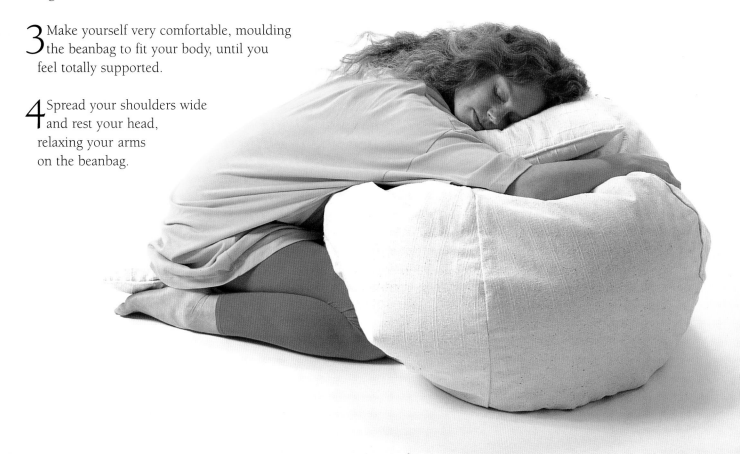

LYING ON YOUR SIDE

While some women find this position very comfortable, others prefer the FRONT SIDE POSITION *opposite. Lying on your left side helps to encourage your baby's spine to the left side of your abdomen, which is the best position for labour. You may wish to vary this by sometimes lying on the right, but it is good to lie often on the left when you rest and sleep, especially in the last six weeks of your pregnancy.*

1 Lie on your left side on a soft surface with your head resting on a cushion. Extend your left leg out behind you and bend the right leg, placing a pillow or two under your right knee.

2 Make sure your arms are positioned comfortably and that your neck and shoulders are relaxed and you can breathe easily.

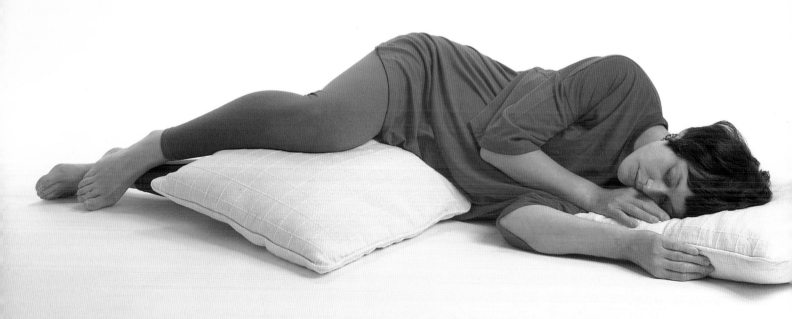

FRONT SIDE POSITION

1 Lie on your left side on a soft surface with your head resting on a cushion. Extend your left leg out behind you and bend the right, placing one or two pillows under the right knee for comfort.

2 Turn your upper body over to face the ground as if you were lying on your front, with your left arm extended downwards behind you and your right arm upwards in front, with your shoulders spread out and relaxed.

3 Rest your head on a small cushion facing your right hand. Make sure you feel completely comfortable.

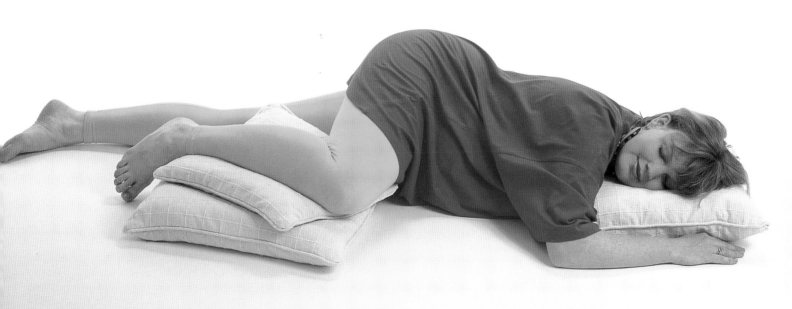

EXERCISING WITH A PARTNER

Working with another person when you exercise is fun. It's a way of involving your partner in your pregnancy with the benefit of helping each other feel relaxed and comfortable in the positions.

All the exercises in this section are designed for two people to do together and, where it is appropriate, taking turns to be the helper and the person exercising You can do them with another pregnant woman, your partner, or a friend or relative. They can also be one in a group or introduced into an antenatal or parenting class, where several pairs work together at the same time.

What you will need

You need the same space and equipment as for 'Exercising on your Own': a simple straightbacked chair and a low stool, some large cushions or a beanbag, small cushions or pillows and a bolster cushion or rolled-up blankets, plus enough clear space to work in. Wear loose comfortable clothing and work on a soft surface – a carpet or folded blankets or use exercise mats.

How to follow the partnerwork instructions

In some exercises, both partners need to follow the same instructions. In others the instructions are different, and here the first set of instructions is meant for you, the pregnant woman, and the second set is for your partner. If you are two pregnant women working together, it is easiest if you decide from the outset who is going to be the 'partner'. Stick to that formula and each follow only those instructions that are meant for you. Then change roles with your partner and repeat the exercise so that you both have a turn before going on to the next one.

Working together

Before doing the exercises it's a good idea to practise the communication exercise, TALKING AND LISTENING (pages 68–69). This is a time to let one another know how each is feeling, how your pregnancy is progressing and what you would each like to achieve in the session. Plan what you would like to do together before you start and keep each other informed about individual needs as the session progresses, as well as letting each other know what feels really good!

Always begin your exercise session by doing some simple BREATHING (see page 12) and end with the RELAXING MASSAGE on page 93. Finish off the session with the BABY AWARENESS exercise on page 91, which can either be done relaxing in your partner's arms (as illustrated) or sitting back-to-back if you are working with a friend. This makes a calm, restful end to your exercise session; alternatively, you can practise it earlier to enhance your awareness of the presence of your baby (or babies) throughout.

When doing the exercises make sure that you are both comfortable. If the instructions suggest touching or massaging your partner, then work gently at first and from time to time check with your partner how it feels.

The massages on page 74–79 and on page 93 and the massages for labour on pages 88–91 can either be done over clothes or directly onto the skin using a light vegetable massage oil, such as almond oil. It is a good idea to warm the oil and pour some into a bowl so that you can use it easily. All the massages are particularly relaxing if given after a warm bath, and will help you to sleep well when done just before you go to bed.

You can also mix the partner sessions with some of the exercises you enjoy from 'Exercising on your Own' if you feel like doing a longer session, but an hour to an hour-and-a-half is long enough at any one time. A session should always end with relaxation and be followed by a drink and perhaps something to eat.

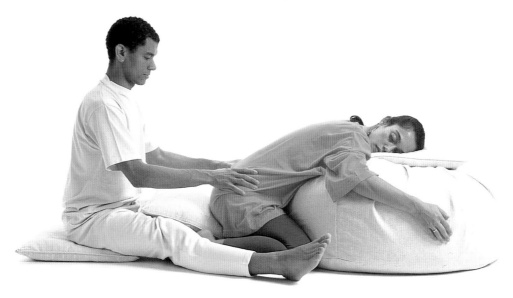

Good communication: 'talking and listening'
Before you begin exercising together, it is always a good idea to set aside a few minutes to practise talking and listening. This exercise is an aid to open communication and will help you to develop the habit of talking about your feelings. It can be done by a couple working together as shown, or you can do it with a friend or relative, or in an antenatal or parenting class. After a while it will seem less like an exercise and will come naturally, enhancing your exercise session as well as your daily life.

Start by sitting down comfortably in one of the easy sitting positions you have learned. Spend three to five minutes doing the breathing exercise on page 12. Then turn to face each other – preferably close enough to touch if you are a couple working together.

In a group or class, divide into pairs and sit at a comfortable distance facing each other, then start by introducing yourself to your partner and telling her a little bit about yourself, your pregnancy and your plans for the birth.

The basic principle of this exercise is that when one person talks, the other listens without interrupting. Allocate a maximum amount of time for speaking – say, between one and five minutes, and then take turns at listening and talking.

It is a good idea to begin by letting your partner know about something you appreciate and feel good about, then go on to say how you are feeling at the moment. Then you can use the time to exchange information, to ask questions, to let your partner know if you have any special request or needs for the exercise session.

For example you might say 'I'm very tired today and all I really want to do is to relax.' Then your partner might respond: 'Thanks for telling me – let's go slowly, and let me know if you want to stop or leave out any of the exercises.'

This simple talking and listening technique can be used in many situations and is especially useful if conflict arises or there is a disagreement in a relationship. If you can develop the habit of sitting down and talking to one another and listening to each other in a calm and balanced way, you will find that most problems can be solved and you can cope with anything that may turn up. It is also a lovely way to share your excitement and pleasures, your wishes, hopes and dreams.

In a group it is an enjoyable way to get to know each other better and to make new friends. You can also use this exercise at home within your family and, later on, it will help you to communicate successfully with your child.

TALKING AND LISTENING

This communication exercise will help you develop the habit of sharing your feelings.

1 Sit on a cushion facing each other with your knees touching and your legs comfortably crossed.

2 Relax your arms and shoulders and rest your hands gently on your partner's knees – or on your own knees, if you prefer, when working with a friend or in a class.

3 In a relaxed way, maintain eye contact as you take turns to talk and listen to each other.

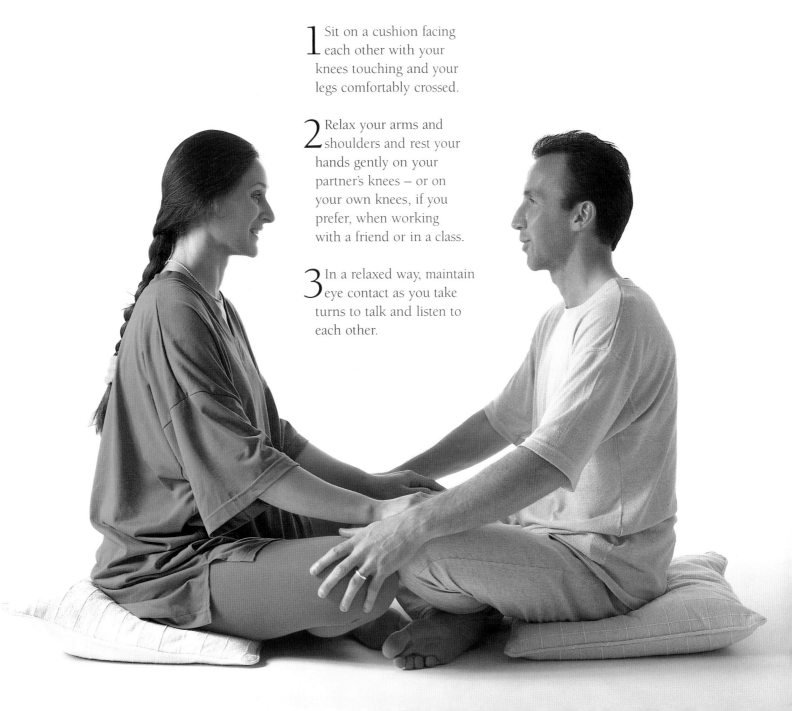

LEGS WIDE – BACK TO BACK

Working together back to back gives you support in the lower back, allowing your pelvis and legs to relax onto the floor with the pull of gravity while your shoulders and spine feel light and free.

1 Sit back to back with your lower backs touching, and spread your legs wide apart to your comfortable limit.

2 Allow your upper back, between the shoulder blades, to make light contact with your partner's, but do not lean on each other heavily.

3 Relax your shoulders and place your hands softly on your thighs.

4 Let your awareness go to your breathing and feel the weight of your pelvis and legs slowly sinking towards the ground with each out breath. Allow your spine to lengthen gently towards the ceiling as you breathe in.

5 Remain in the position for up to three minutes or until one of you wants to stop.

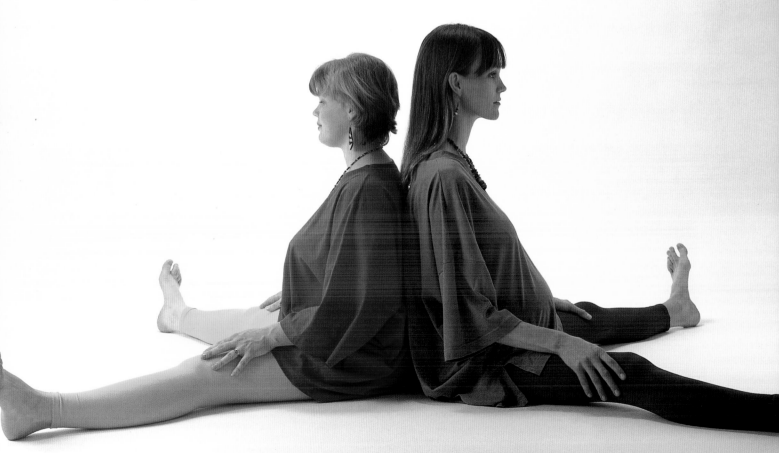

LEGS WIDE – FEET IN THE BACK

Some people find this more comfortable than the exercise opposite, and it supports your lower back in a similar way.

1 Sit with your legs spread wide apart and let your partner's feet support your lower back.

2 Relax in the position for a minute or so, releasing the back of your neck by tilting your head slightly forwards.

3 Continue focusing on the natural flow of your breathing.

4 To come out of the position, slowly bring your legs together with the help of your hands, and then move away from your partner.

Partner

1 Place the soles of your feet firmly against your partner's lower back.

2 Straighten your legs and lean back slightly, supporting yourself with your hands. Keep your shoulders relaxed and make sure that you feel comfortable.

3 Breathing evenly, gently increase the pressure of your feet until your partner feels well supported.

4 Focus on your breathing and the downward pull of gravity through your legs.

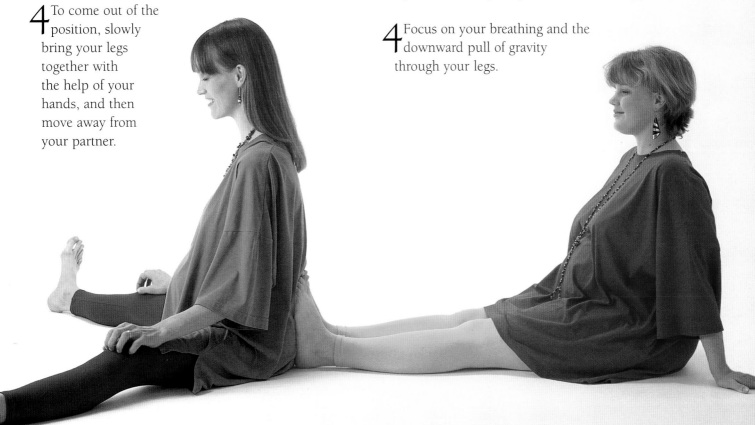

TAILOR SITTING – BACK TO BACK

This is a warm friendly way to practise tailor sitting with your back supported comfortably.

1 Bring your lower back as close to your partner's as possible.

2 Bend your knees and place the soles of your feet together at a comfortable distance from your body.

3 Place a cushion or two under your knees so that your legs are well supported and you can relax.

4 Relax your shoulders and feel your upper back making gentle contact with your partner. Relax your arms and place your hands on your calves.

5 Now close your eyes and focus on your breathing. Feel your lower back and hips release towards the floor while your spine lengthens from the back of your waist up towards the top of your neck.

Remember

Avoid leaning heavily against your partner, bouncing your knees or pulling your legs in too close to your body.

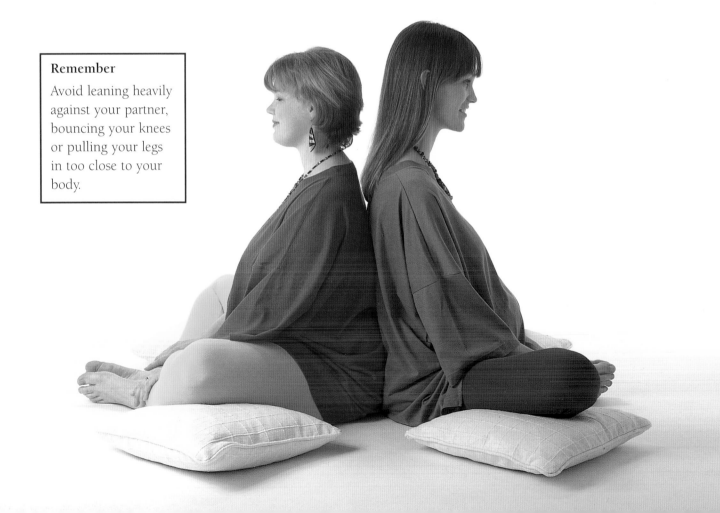

TAILOR SITTING – FEET IN THE BACK

This is a very comfortable way to be supported while tailor sitting.

1 Bend your knees and place the soles of your feet together at a comfortable distance from your body.

2 Use cushions to support your legs unless they rest comfortably on the ground

3 Relax and focus on the wave of your breathing for a minute or two.

Partner

1 Place the soles of both feet firmly against the lower back.

2 Straighten your legs and lean back slightly, supporting yourself with your hands.

3 Breathe evenly and increase the pressure gently until your partner feels well supported.

4 Focus on your breathing and the downward pull of gravity through your legs.

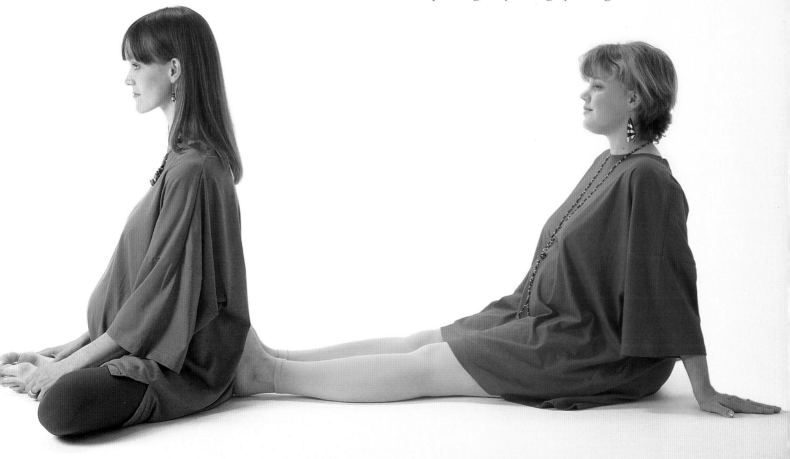

KNEELING

SHOULDER MASSAGE

The exercises on pages 74–79 can be done as one massage sequence. Practise all of them on a soft surface suitable for kneeling, and use a long cushion or bolster, plus several small cushions if necessary, so that your hips are raised a little higher than your knees and are well supported throughout. Place a beanbag and cushion in front of you, ready for leaning forwards later on.

1 Kneel in UPRIGHT CHILD'S POSE (page 32) and relax. Close your eyes and focus your awareness on your breathing.

2 Release your lower back downwards, following the curve of the bones at the base of your spine. Feel your weight settle in your pelvis.

3 Gently lengthen your spine towards the top of your neck and release your chin downwards slightly. Relax your jaw and your shoulders as your partner begins the massage.

Partner

1 Place a cushion on a low stool and sit comfortably behind your partner. Place your hands gently on the shoulders.

2 Focus on your breathing and notice how the muscles feel under your hands.

3 Massage the shoulders with a relaxed kneading movement, checking how much pressure feels comfortable.

4 Continue for a minute or two, working gently into the neck and the base of the skull, then down into the upper back, around the shoulder blades and down the arms.

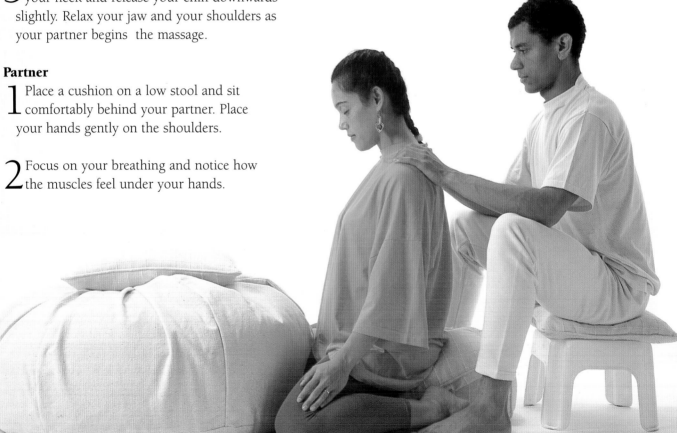

LOWER BACK RELEASE

This movement keeps the pelvis well grounded, allowing the spine to lengthen as the shoulders release and the arms come up.

1 Be aware of your breathing and release your lower back downwards.

2 As your partner holds your hips, slowly raise both arms up over your head, keeping your elbows slightly bent and your shoulders down.

3 Hold the position for a few moments and then slowly lower your arms.

Partner

1 Sit on the floor behind your partner on a small cushion with your legs apart so that you feel comfortable and relaxed.

2 Place your hands around the pelvic bones so that they rest securely on the rim.

3 Exert a continuous gentle downward pressure to encourage the pelvis to relax downwards with the pull of gravity.

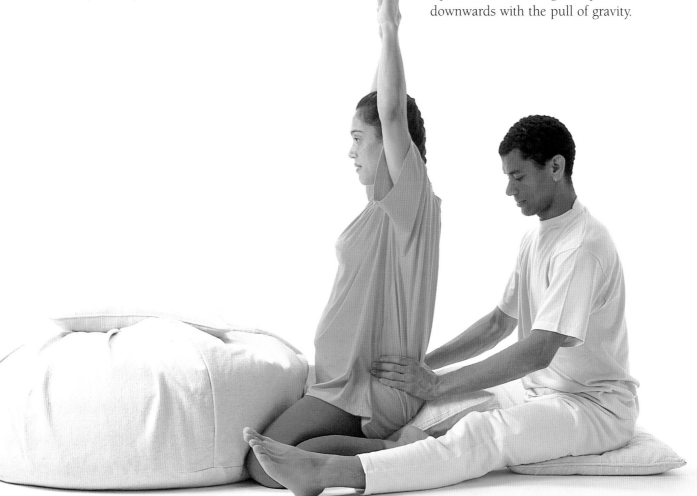

LOWER BACK MASSAGE

Leaning forwards onto a beanbag takes the weight off your lower back and is a perfect position for a massage. While you are relaxing, this position is also helping to guide your baby into a good position for the birth and releasing tension in the groin, hips, knees and ankles.

1 Lean forwards slowly, moving from your hips, and relax onto the beanbag with your upper body comfortably supported.

2 Turn your head to one side and rest it on the beanbag, with your neck relaxed and eyes closed. Relax your shoulders and spread your arms out loosely to the sides.

3 Focus your awareness on your breathing and let go completely, allowing yourself to sink into a peaceful relaxation as your partner works.

Partner

1 Gently hold the pelvis down as your partner moves forwards.

2 Place both hands over the lower back and pause for a moment or two, focusing on your breathing and the sensations in your hands.

3 Once your partner is relaxed and comfortable, begin to work with your thumbs, massaging over the pelvic bones.

4 Then use both hands to circle up the centre of the lower back and then around the sides, including the hips and buttocks.

5 Continue like this for a minute or two, making smooth, soothing movements.

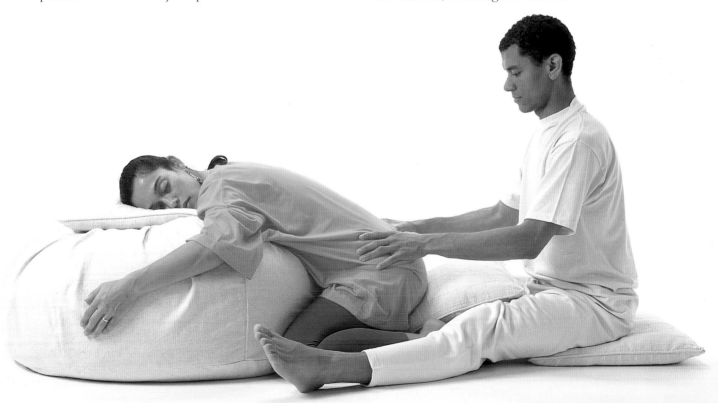

LONG STROKES

These strokes relax the long muscles that run down either side of the spine, and move the energy from the head and shoulders down towards the pelvis, helping to release tension in the upper body.

1 Rest on the beanbag as shown opposite and continue breathing and relaxing while your partner works.

Partner

1 Kneel with one knee on a cushion and the other one raised so that you are comfortable.

2 Using one hand and then the other in a smooth alternating rhythm, stroke down the spine from the neck to the tailbone.

3 Continue for a minute or so, stroking slowly and softly, and end by resting both hands on the lower back.

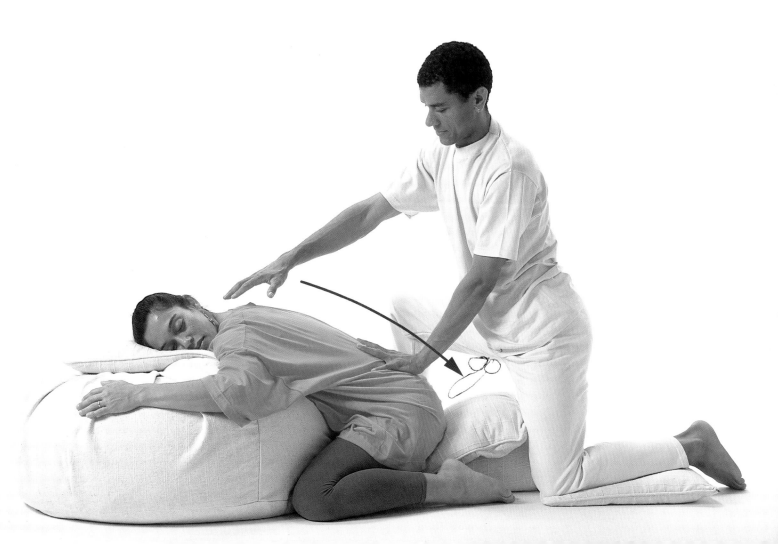

FULL BODY STROKES

This wonderful massage stroke was invented by a father I taught many years ago, who used it throughout labour to 'take away the pain'. In pregnancy, it is very comforting and relaxing, clearing the energy, releasing tension and tiredness from the whole body through the feet.

1 Rest on a beanbag as on page 76 and continue breathing and relaxing while your partner works.

Partner

1 Kneel as shown on page 77 and, using your left hand only, start at the left shoulder, placing your palm flat with fingers relaxed.

2 Beginning as your partner exhales, stroke slowly down the left side of the spine. In one continuous movement, go around the left hip, along the thigh, around the knee, along the calf and out through the toes.

3 Flick your hand to discharge the energy, then repeat the same movement with the right hand on the right side.

4 Continue alternating left and right sides until you have done three strokes on each side, and then repeat the movement three times with both hands down both sides simultaneously.

5 Repeat this whole sequence two or three times, and end by resting both hands on the lower back.

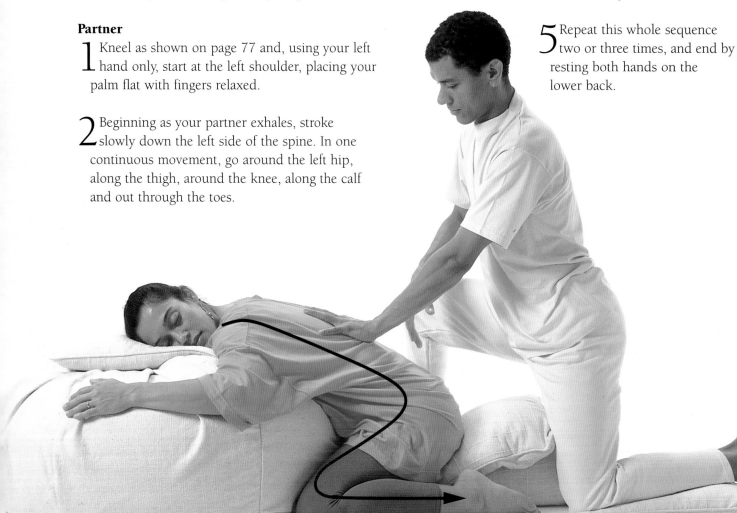

COMING UP SLOWLY

Returning to the vertical position slowly like this allows the weight to first settle in the pelvis and the heavy base of the spine before the rest of the spine lengthens gradually upwards towards the neck. This creates a feeling of relaxation and release in the neck and shoulders and a sense of lightness in the upper body.

1 Let your awareness go down into your pelvis. Breathe evenly as you begin to release the curve of your lower back downwards with the help of your partner.

2 Curl up to the vertical position, starting from the base and working slowly upwards so that your shoulders, neck and head come up last.

Partner

1 Sit or kneel down comfortably behind your partner and place both hands firmly over the base of the spine.

2 Exert a gentle downward pressure as your partner begins to come up, to encourage the lower back to drop first, and then stroke down the spine as it lengthens.

3 Once the spine is vertical, remove your hands and end with a brief massage of the shoulders and down the arms.

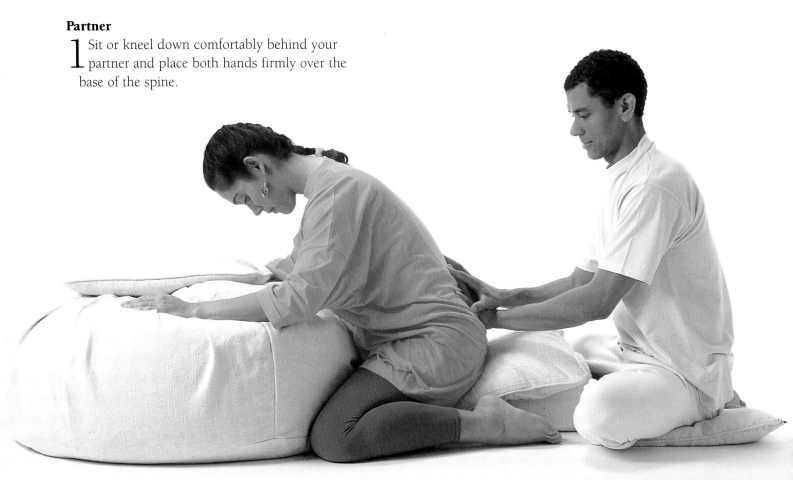

GROUNDING

Working with a partner while doing this exercise helps you to surrender to the pull of gravity coming from the ground. Your body feels well grounded from the feet up to the waist, while the upper body responds by relaxing as tension releases from the neck and shoulders. This helps to develop good postural awareness when standing and walking.

1 Stand with your feet about 30cm/12in (hip's width) apart, with your heels slightly wider apart than your toes.

2 As your partner helps, be aware of your breathing and relax the soles of your feet, sensing the ground underneath you.

3 Feel your weight fall evenly through both heels and release your lower back downwards.

Partner

1 Kneel or sit on the floor behind your partner and hold both of the heels, exerting a downward pressure.

2 Hold for a few moments and then, using both hands, stroke down the lower back, through the hips and down the back of the legs, through the heels into the floor in one continuous movement. Repeat this five or six times.

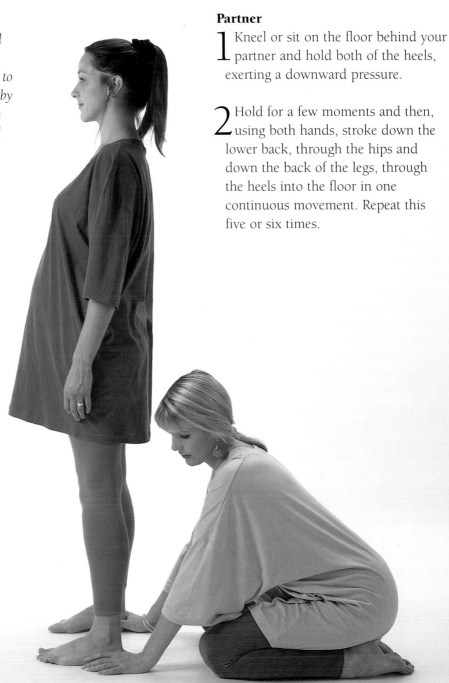

BENDING FORWARDS

This forward bend releases tension in the hamstring muscles at the back of the legs,
and also lengthens the spine and relaxes the shoulders.

Remember

Leave this one out if
you feel uncomfortable
or light-headed when
you bend forwards, or
if you have painful
haemorrhoids.

1 Stand as for GROUNDING opposite, facing your
partner. Keep your weight dropping through
your heels and lean forwards slowly from your
hips until your trunk is parallel to the floor.

2 Extend both arms with elbows straight, and
as your partner supports you, relax your
shoulders and gently lengthen your spine.
Keep dropping your weight through your
heels and breathe evenly.

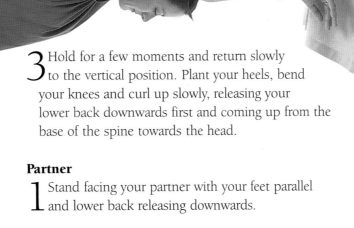

3 Hold for a few moments and return slowly
to the vertical position. Plant your heels, bend
your knees and curl up slowly, releasing your
lower back downwards first and coming up from the
base of the spine towards the head.

Partner

1 Stand facing your partner with your feet parallel
and lower back releasing downwards.

2 When she bends forwards, support her wrists softly
from underneath without bending your
own back or leaning forwards.

CALF STRETCH

This exercise lengthens the calf muscles and the back of the heels, helping to increase flexibility in the ankles. This makes squatting easier and can also relieve cramps in the calves.

1 Stand facing a wall in the STANDING WELL or GROUNDING positions (pages 40 or 80) at an arm's distance from the wall.

2 Place your right leg forwards with the knee bent and your left leg back with the knee straight and heel down on the ground. Both feet remain parallel.

3 Keeping your hips in line with the wall, link your hands and lean forwards onto your forearms and elbows, with neck and shoulders relaxed. Breathe evenly, feeling the stretch in the back of your left leg.

4 Hold for three cycles of the breath and then change to the other side. Repeat on both legs twice.

Partner

1 Kneel or sit comfortably behind your partner.

2 Use your left hand to ground the heel, pressing down gently but firmly. Your right hand supports the front of the knee, gently encouraging the back of the leg to open.

3 Hold until your partner changes legs, then repeat on the other side reversing your hand positions.

SUPPORTING FROM BEHIND

Practising your squatting regularly will help you to be at ease in supported squat positions during labour and birth by slowly increasing the flexibility of your hips, knees and ankles and strengthening your thighs.

1 Place your feet a little wider apart than your normal standing position and slightly turned out. Position a bolster, pile of books or low stool between your legs. Breathe evenly.

2 With your partner behind you, bend your knees and, keeping both heels down on the floor, slowly lower your pelvis into the squatting position.

3 Hold for a minute or two and then come up by pressing your heels down, slowly raising your pelvis and straightening your legs. Alternatively you can come forwards onto your hands and knees before coming up. Repeat once or twice more.

Partner

1 Stand behind your partner so that her lower back is supported by your legs. Breathe evenly.

2 Bend forwards from your hips, keeping your own back relaxed and place your hands on your partner's knees. Relax your neck and shoulders and lean softly down onto the knees to create a gentle sense of downward pressure towards your partner's heels.

3 To assist your partner coming up, support the rib cage gently on both sides, just under the arms with your hands.

Remember

Avoid deep squats in the last six weeks of pregnancy. Leave out the partner squats on pages 83–85 until your midwife or doctor has confirmed that your baby's head has fully engaged.

If you have weak or painful knees, use a low stool under your pelvis and avoid deep squats.

PARTNER ON A CHAIR

This is an easy way to practise squatting and can also be used occasionally during labour to strengthen contractions or as a birthing position.

1 Stand facing your partner with your feet wider apart than your usual standing position and slightly turned out, holding each other by the wrists so that both of you have your arms outstretched.

2 Breathe evenly and, keeping your heels on the floor, bend your knees and slowly lower your pelvis until your buttocks rest on the support. Make sure that you are the right distance from your partner so that both of you can keep your arms straight.

3 Relax and lengthen your back and neck and hold for three to five cycles of the breathing rhythm. Stand up slowly by planting your heels down, slowly raising your pelvis and straightening your legs. Repeat this twice more.

Partner

1 Hold your partner by the wrists and sit down securely on a chair with your feet well grounded and knees comfortably apart. Relax your lower back towards the seat of the chair and breathe evenly.

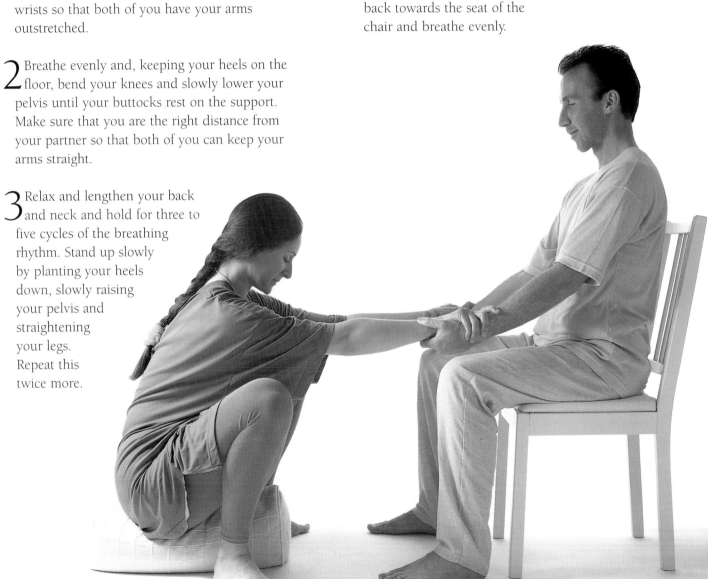

SQUATTING TOGETHER

This way of practising squatting is more challenging, so leave it out if you find squatting difficult. You can also make it easier with both or one of you using the support of a bolster or stool.

1 Stand facing each other and hold each other firmly by the wrists with arms outstretched and elbows straight. Place your feet a little wider apart than your usual standing position and slightly turned out.

2 Keeping your heels down, breathe evenly and, moving together, slowly bend your knees and lower your pelvis into a squat. Make sure that you are far enough away from your partner to pull gently on each other for support with your back relaxed, heels down and arms straight.

3 Hold for a short while and then come up together slowly, still holding on. As you come up, press your heels down into the ground, gently raise your pelvis and slowly straighten your legs. Rest and then repeat twice more.

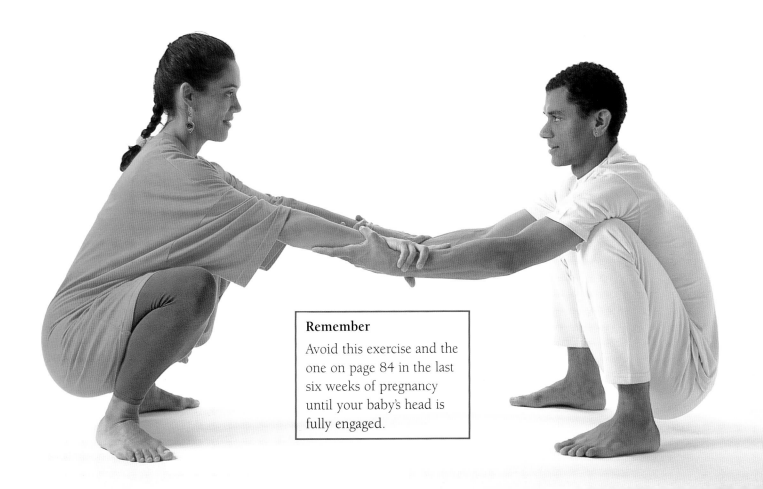

Remember
Avoid this exercise and the one on page 84 in the last six weeks of pregnancy until your baby's head is fully engaged.

MASSAGE FOR LABOUR

You may be planning to share your labour with a partner. If so it's a good idea to do some practising together throughout your pregnancy – and especially in the last six weeks.

The following exercises involve massage and can be practised over clothes. Sometimes, however, it is helpful and enjoyable to work directly on the skin using a mild vegetable massage oil. This will prepare you for working in labour, when the skin may become irritated by massage over clothing; in this case it is better to work with oil on the skin.

Preparing for massage

Create an atmosphere in which you both feel comfortable, with low lighting or candlelight and perhaps some soothing music in the background, at a time when you won't be interrupted. Make sure the room is warm – though not too warm – and pleasant to be in. You can do this session at any time but it's especially enjoyable after a bath before going to bed.

Start by spending 10 minutes doing the breathing and baby awareness exercises together (see pages 12, 13 and 92).

Tune in to the presence of your baby so that you are conscious of your child being there with you throughout. It is as important to be able to be silent and peaceful together, without doing anything else, as it is to do practical things, so take your time before you start.

Massage in pregnancy

The exercises that follow suggest some simple massage techniques which can be used in labour. Many women find that massage in labour is helpful for comfort and pain relief, while others prefer not to be touched. It is impossible to predict whether this sort of help will be useful at the time. However, most women find massage enjoyable in late pregnancy and it is worth doing now, even if in labour you decide you don't want to be massaged. Massage helps you to develop the art of communicating through touch and will enhance your relationship. Once you get used to being massaged in kneeling or standing positions, try alternatives such as sitting astride a chair facing backwards, resting your upper body, arms and head on a pillow, or kneeling over a beanbag.

The massaging partner

If you are the partner giving the massage, it is important for you to be comfortable as well. Wear light comfortable clothing and, if it helps you feel more at ease, do use a low stool, some cushions or a bolster to sit on as you work.

Make sure your arms and shoulders are relaxed, your back feels loose and comfortable, and your hands are warm. Take your time before starting to massage your partner. First focus on your own breathing and notice how your body feels. Then pause to release any tension that you have become aware of in your neck, shoulders, arms or legs.

When you are ready, bring your hands into contact with her body very slowly, and start the massage gently, asking her after a while how it feels, whether she would like more or less pressure and whether your hands are in the right place. You will find, in time, that these sessions are so enjoyable that you will soon become a confident and intuitive masseur, developing your own style and method of helping your partner with a touch that is sensitive to her needs at the time.

Keep it simple and relaxed, thinking in your mind of soothing movements that help to take away pain. You will notice that these massage strokes focus on the lower back. This is because the sacral nerves from the uterus go up through the lower back into the spinal cord towards the brain. When you massage this area during a contraction in labour the pleasant sensations you are creating travel to the brain and help to influence your partner's perception of the pain in a positive way. However, if you notice that her shoulders look tense then use your intuition and work for a while on her shoulders, or try the full body strokes on page 78, using oil on the skin.

It is usually best to massage during the contractions, and to stop in between them to rest.

Sharing your feelings

When you practise, change over from time to time and let your partner receive a massage too. This is a creative way to exchange ideas and information about ways you like to be touched. It is a good idea to complete your massage session with the TALKING AND LISTENING exercise on page 69. Start by telling each other all the things you appreciated about the massage – what felt good! Then take turns to share information about anything you would like to be different next time and recommend specifically how you would like your partner to work – ideally with a demonstration. End by thanking each other and planning a time for your next practice session. You may also like to go on to practise the relaxation exercises on pages 92 and 93.

CIRCLING

1 Kneel on a soft surface in the all-fours position or over a beanbag. Make sure your neck and shoulders are relaxed and that there is no discomfort in your wrists.

2 Breathe in through your nose and out slowly through your mouth, as if you were in labour, while moving your body or circling your hips rhythmically as your partner is working.

3 Continue for a minute or two and come up slowly when you are ready. Rest and then repeat once or twice

Partner

1 Kneel comfortably behind your partner or sit on a stool for support. Place both hands gently on her lower back and breathe evenly, relaxing your hands.

2 Slowly make a circular movement with both hands, stroking up the lower back towards the waistline and then around the hips and back to the centre. Continue like this for a minute or two with a smooth even pressure.

3 Now try using one hand only to make a broader circle around the whole of the lower back and hips. Continue until your partner is ready to come up.

4 Repeat both of these massage strokes once more, but remember to ask first how it felt.

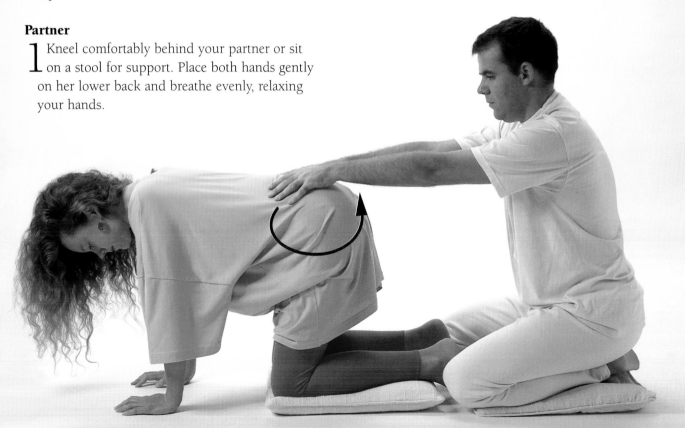

BASE OF THE SPINE

1 Kneel on a soft surface in the all-fours position or over a beanbag. Make sure your neck and shoulders are released and that there is no discomfort in your wrists.

2 Lean backwards towards your partner's hand using the pressure to create a gentle sense of resistance. This may help to relieve pain during contractions in labour.

3 Continue for a minute or so and then come up.

Partner

1 Kneel behind your partner with one leg raised and place the palm of one hand over the lower back so that the tailbone is just below the heel of your palm.

2 Keep your elbow straight and gently lean your body weight towards your hand, providing an even pressure for your partner to lean into.

3 Allow your partner to move and do the work while you simply offer gentle resistance.

4 Keep your hand in position for a moment or two and then rest.

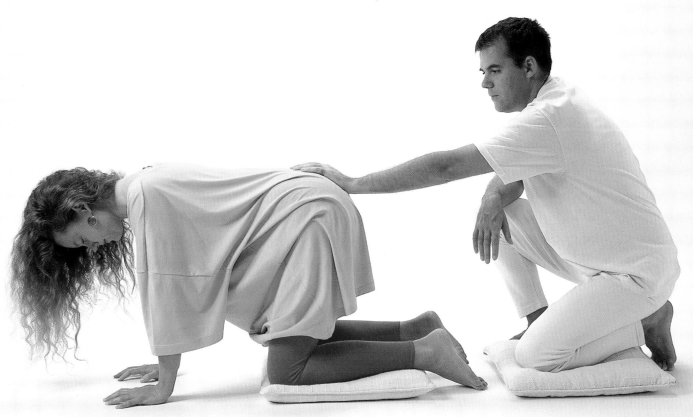

CIRCLING THE HIPS

1 Stand comfortably facing a wall. Fold your arms and place them on the wall, resting your head on your forearms with neck and shoulders relaxed.

2 Breathe in through your nose and out through your mouth and slowly rotate your hips as you may like to do in labour.

3 Let your partner know how the massage feels or if you would like more pressure.

Partner

1 Stand comfortably beside your partner and rest the palm of one hand in the centre of her lower back at the height of the waistline. Relax your arm and breathe evenly.

2 Tune in to her movements and then slowly massage down and around her lower back and hips using a slow continuous circular movement. Keep the pressure soft and even unless she asks you to massage more firmly.

3 Continue for a minute or so and then rest. Repeat once or twice.

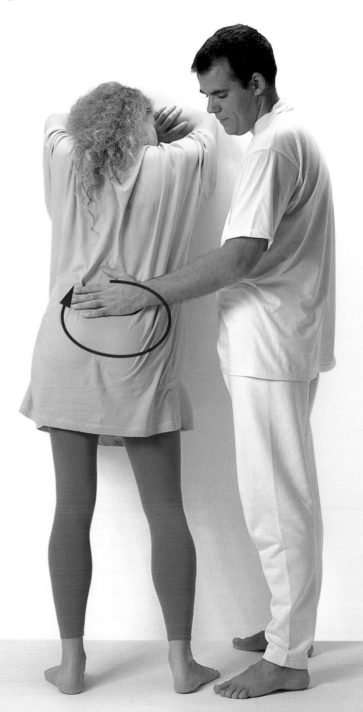

SIDE TO SIDE

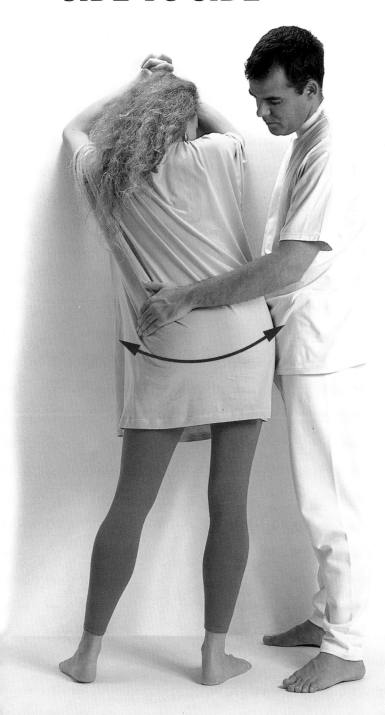

1 Stand comfortably facing a wall. Clasp your hands or fold your arms and place them on the wall, resting your head against them with neck and shoulders relaxed.

2 Swing your hips from side to side while breathing evenly.

3 Let your partner know how the massage feels.

Partner

1 Stand to the side of your partner with your hand resting gently on her hip and focus on your own breathing for a few seconds.

2 Tune in to her movements and then stroke across her lower back. Work in the opposite direction to her movements so that as she comes towards you, your hand moves away, and as she moves away, your hand comes back towards you.

3 Continue for a minute or so and then rest and repeat once or twice.

BABY AWARENESS

Tuning in to the presence of your baby creates a feeling of peace and harmony – a perfect way to end the exercise session before relaxation or to use before you begin working together. It is especially pleasurable to share the baby awareness exercise with your partner, giving him and your baby an opportunity to begin to get to know each other before the birth.

1 Make sure you are completely comfortable, lying in your partner's arms with your back supported. If you are working with another pregnant mother, sit back to back so that your lower backs are in contact and your spine feels free; fold your legs comfortably with cushions under your knees. Close your eyes and let your hands rest softly on your partner's hands or your belly.

2 Let your awareness go to your breathing. Exhaling and inhaling in a comfortable rhythm, let any feelings of tension or tightness in your body melt away. Feel your whole body becoming softer and more relaxed with each breath. Continue exactly as for the BABY AWARENESS exercise on page 13.

Partner

1 If you are holding your partner, sit on a cushion with your back well supported against a wall. Support your partner as she leans against you, making sure you are both comfortable.

2 Bring your awareness to the presence of your baby and try communicating with your baby by stroking your partner's belly with your hands or visualizing and 'talking' inwardly to your baby.

3 Spend a minute or so resting and relaxing with your baby and then very slowly bring your awareness back to your breathing, your body and the room around you. Open your eyes and relax.

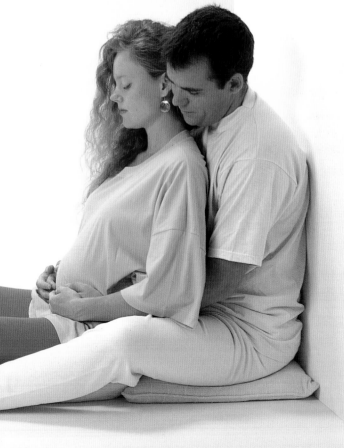

RELAXING MASSAGE

This is a wonderful way to end your session of exercising together. When done in a group or by two pregnant mothers working together, one begins massaging the other and then they swap over. A couple can use this after a warm bath in the evening, to help the pregnant mother have a peaceful sleep.

1 Lie on your right side first, with a cushion under your head and one or two cushions supporting your left leg. Make sure that you are completely comfortable. Relax and breathe evenly, letting go of all thoughts.

2 Let your body surrender to the support of the ground and the touch of your partner's hands, releasing and relaxing as you breathe.

3 Turn over when your partner has finished massaging the left side.

Partner

1 Kneel comfortably behind your partner and place one hand on her hip and the other around the top of her shoulder. Massage into the shoulder, around the shoulder blade and the side of the neck, encouraging the muscles to relax and release.

2 Work down the top arm and along the forearm to the hand. Then work slowly down the back along the spine, pausing to work into any area that feels tight or tense.

3 Work down through the waistline to the lower back. Focus on the uppermost side of the lower back and the top hip and then continue down the top leg and foot to the toes.

4 Ask your partner to turn over onto the left side and repeat the massage down the right side of her body.

5 Cover your partner with something warm to rest for a few minutes before you change over, or to sleep if you are doing this at bedtime.

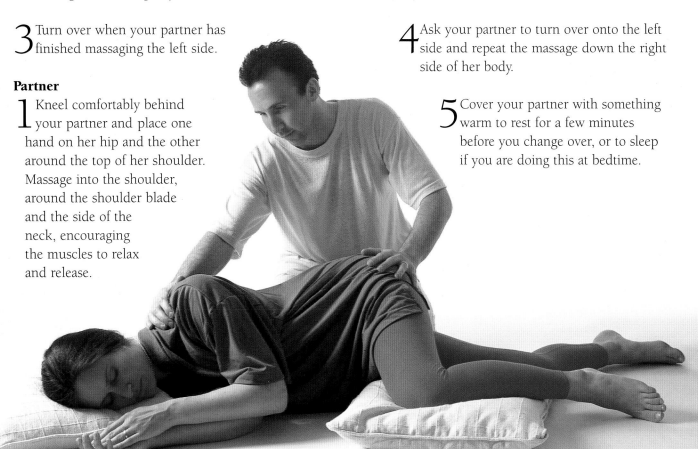

INDEX

S

sciatica, 11
shoulders: massage, 74
  shoulder release, 17, 20
  shoulder stretch, 21
side, lying on, 64
side to side massage, 91
sitting positions:
  legs wide - back to back, 70
  legs wide - feet in the back, 71
  legs wide leaning back, 28
  sitting well, 30-1
  tailor position, 26-7
  tailor sitting - back to back, 72
  tailor sitting - feet in the back, 73

tailor sitting leaning back, 29
spine see back
spreading out, 22
squatting, 8
  full squat, 46-7
  holding on, 45
  labour positions, 59
  partner on a chair, 84
  squatting together, 85
  supporting from behind, 83
  using a stool, 44
standing, 40
  labour positions, 57
stools, squatting, 44
suppleness, 7-8

T

tailor position, 26-7
  back to back, 72
  feet in the back, 73
  leaning back, 29
talking, partnerwork, 68-9
tiredness, 7
toes and heels, 14
twists: gentle sitting twist, 23
  gentle standing twist, 42

U

upright child's pose, 32

Useful addresses

The Active Birth Centre
25 Bickerton Road
London N19 5JT
Tel: 0171 561 9006
Fax: 0171 561 9007
Directed by Janet Balaskas, the Active Birth
Centre offers classes in this system of exercises
as well as a register of teachers throughout the
U.K. and in many other countries. They are
also a resource centre for water birth and
birth pool hire and have a mail order
catalogue of books and aromatherapy
products, including massage oils specifically
for labour and birth.

Cranial Osteopathic Association Ltd
478 Baker Street
Enfield
Middlesex EN1 3QS
Tel: 0181 367 5561

General Council and Register
of Osteopaths
56 London Street
Reading
RG1 4SQ
Tel: 01734 576585

National Childbirth Trust (NCT)
Alexandra House
Oldham Terrace
London W3 6NH
Tel: 0181 992 8637

Osteopathy Pregnancy Clinic
The British School of Osteopathy
Littlejohn House
1-4 Suffolk Street
London SW1 4HG
Tel: 0171 930 9254

Further reading

Other useful works by Janet Balaskas that
complement the pregnancy exercise system
she has devised and reflect her approach
to preparing for birth include: *Active Birth*
(Thorsons), *The Encyclopedia of Pregnancy*
and Birth, co-author Yehudi Gordon (Little,
Brown), *Natural Pregnancy* (Gaia Books),
Water Birth, co-author Yehudi Gordon
(Thorsons), *Preparing for Birth with Yoga*
(Element), and the videos *Active Birth*,
Water Birth and the audio casstette *Yoga for*
Pregnancy (all Active Birth Centre
Publications).

Author's Acknowledgments

I would like to thank Sylvia Bazzarelli and Marcus Dos Santos, Sarah Boyce, Naoko Chalkley, Jo Hamilton, Clare Harrison, Maureen Hibbert, Francesca Iliffe and Stephen Miller, Laila Mastenbrook, Julie Ann Miller, Harriet Mould, Juliette and Alan Stuart, Michelle Twiddy, Adrienne Wilkinson – the pregnant mothers and their partners from my classes who cheerfully posed for the lovely pictures which illustrate this book – and also Anthea Sieveking who photographed them so beautifully. Thanks also to my colleagues and fellow Active Birth Teachers who have participated in the evolution of the exercises, refining them with the benefit of our shared experience. I am also very grateful to Jean Sutton for her work on 'Optimal Foetal Positioning' which has enabled me to revise and update the exercises so that pregnant mothers can use their bodies sensibly to encourage a problem-free and normal childbirth. Judy Hargreaves has inspired me to introduce the communication exercises for partners to do together into this programme with her wonderful work with couples and families. Thanks also go to Bumblebee for the loan of clothes for photography. This is my first book published by Frances Lincoln and I would like to thank everyone involved for making the creation of this book such an enjoyable experience.

Publishers' Acknowledgments

Editors Sarah Mitchell
       Alison Freegard
Art editor Louise Kirby
Initial design Sally Cracknell
Designer Sara Robin
Editorial assistant Jon Folland
Production Jennifer Cohen
Index Hilary Bird

Editorial Director Erica Hunningher
Art Director Caroline Hillier

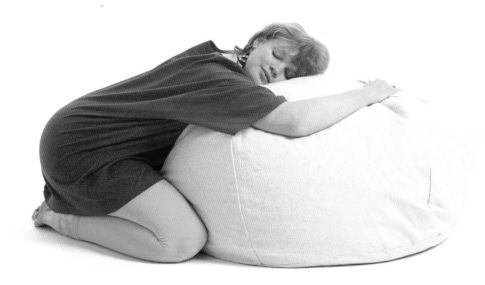